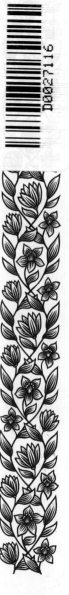

# Llewellyn's
# *Herbal*
# *Almanac*
## *2013*

Cover Design: Kevin R. Brown

Cover Images:
Basil: iStockphoto.com/Olga Weber
White rose: iStockphoto.com/Tathagata Mandal
Butterfly: iStockphoto.com/cyfrogclone
Garlic: iStockphoto.com/Eleonora Ivanova
Bee: iStockphoto.com/Mervana
Jalapeno pepper: iStockphoto.com/dondesigns
Herbs: iStockphoto.com/pinkcoala
Mint: iStockphoto.com/Victoria Ryabinina
Pink rose and leaves: iStockphoto.com/Lee Pettet

Interior Art: © Fiona King

You can order annuals and books from *New
Worlds*, Llewellyn's catalog. To request a free
copy, call toll free: 1-877-NEW WRLD or
visit http://www.llewellyn.com.

ISBN 978-0-7387-1516-2
Llewellyn Worldwide Ltd.
2143 Wooddale Drive
Woodbury, MN 55125-2989

# Contents

## Growing and Gathering Herbs

## Culinary Herbs

## Herbs for Health and Beauty

## Herb Crafts

## Herb History, Myth, and Lore

# Moon Signs, Phases, and Tables

# Introduction to Llewellyn's
# Herbal Almanac

More and more people are using herbs, growing and gathering them, and studying them for their enlivening and healing properties. In the 2013 edition of the *Herbal Almanac*, we pay tribute to the ideals of beauty and balance in relation to the health-giving and beautifying properties of herbs. Whether it comes in the form of a natural herbal bath, a delightful moon garden, or a new favorite recipe, herbs can clearly make a positive impact in your life.

This year we once again bring to these pages some of the most innovative and original thinkers and writers on herbs. We tap into practical, historical, and just plain enjoyable aspects of herbal knowledge—using herbs to help you reconnect with the earth, attract wildlife to your garden, enhance your culinary creations, and heal your body and mind. The thirty-one articles in this almanac will teach you everything from how to plant an herb garden to how to craft the perfect carrier oils for your herbs. Enjoy!

Note: The old-fashioned remedies in this book are historical references used for teaching purposes only. The recipes are not for commercial use or profit. The contents are not meant to diagnose, treat, prescribe, or substitute consultation with a licensed health-care professional. Herbs, whether used internally or externally, should be introduced in small amounts to allow the body to adjust and to detect possible allergies. Please consult a standard reference source or an expert herbalist to learn more about the possible effects of certain herbs. You must take care not to replace regular medical treatment with the use of herbs. Herbal treatment is intended primarily to complement modern health care. Always seek professional help if you suffer from illness. Also, take care to read all warning labels before taking any herbs or starting on an extended herbal regimen. Always consult medical and herbal professionals before beginning any sort of medical treatment—this is particularly true for pregnant women. Herbs are powerful things; be sure you are using that power to achieve balance.

Llewellyn Worldwide does not participate in, endorse, or have any authority or responsibility concerning private business transactions between its authors and the public.

# Growing
# and
# Gathering
# Herbs

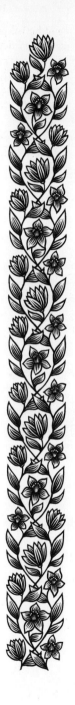

# Early Season Gardening with Herbs

### ⚘ By Elizabeth Barrette ⚘

A garden begins long before sum-mer turns the world green. One of the best times to plan a new garden, or the expansion and refinement of an established garden, is during the winter. You can order your seeds and plants in advance, both for old and new gardens. Some herbs lend them-selves well to starting indoors for later transplant. Then in early spring, you can prepare the garden space itself so it will be ready to receive your herbs when the weather warms up enough.

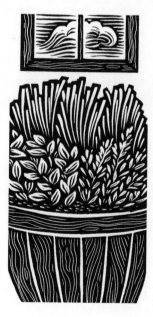

## Garden Design

Unlike vegetable gardens, which tend to take up substantial space, herb gar-dens tend toward a smaller scale. This makes them ideal for balconies, patios, and urban yards. Even in large rural yards, the herb garden is often a little pocket garden right next to the house. Several designs in particular work well with this aspect of herb gardening. Plan an herb garden anytime in winter and set it up in early spring. Prepare and enrich the soil before sowing seeds or transplanting seedlings in mid- to late spring.

On the smallest end of the spectrum, you can grow an herb garden in a single container. Two excellent choices are the strawberry pot and the barrel garden. Choose the strawberry pot if you like both upright and trailing herbs; you plant the upright ones in the large upper hole and the trailing ones in the small side holes. For instance, you might fill the top with French sorrel, sage, and tarragon, while the side pockets hold chamomile, Mother-of-thyme, oregano, prostrate rosemary, trailing nasturtium, and Corsican mint. In a barrel garden you could choose basil, chives, cilantro, Italian parsley, sweet marjoram, and summer and winter savory.

Moving up a step are container gardens featuring a multitude of pots. Shopping before the main garden season can turn up bargains on containers that would be much more expensive at peak demand. Container gardens are adaptable because you can always add or rearrange pots as needed. This approach is ideal if you want to grow herbs that try to take over the world, such as most varieties of mint. It's also good for separating herbs that shouldn't grow too close together, such as plain chives and garlic chives or dill and fennel. Many container gardens live on a porch or patio rather than bare earth. You can even fasten containers to a wall, taking up no ground space at all!

Moving a little outward, we find designs intended to pack herbs into a concise space suitable for a dooryard garden. Two popular choices here are the herb spiral and the keyhole bed. An herb spiral begins at ground level, then slopes upward, ending at about waist height, with a spiral path of flat stones helping to hold the earth in place. This works well with Mediterranean herbs that prefer dry soil with sand or gravel; if you're in a damp climate or have clay soil, this will let you grow different plants. A keyhole garden is basically a round garden with a path leading to a small circle in the center. This design allows you to harvest herbs from both the inside and the outside. Ideally, face the path southward to catch the sun, and plant with shorter plants on the inner circle and taller plants along the outer edge.

## Herb Suppliers

There are many different places to obtain herbs, either as seeds or as plants. Take care when choosing a supplier. You may want organic herbs, or open-pollinated "heritage" or "antique" varieties rather than hybrids. At a minimum, make sure the herbs are sustainably produced and not harmfully (perhaps illegally) removed from the wild.

Early in the season, in winter, you can browse mail-order catalogs either in print or online. Thinking about green growing things can help dispel the gloom of the cold, dark season. Place your order when convenient for you, then the company will ship your herbs at the right time for planting in your area. Large garden companies may carry some herbs, usually the common culinary ones. However, for rarer magical or medicinal herbs, you probably need to find a specialty herb catalog.

Compare different places to find the best selection and pricing. Here are some suppliers to get you started.

## Burpee

Burpee offers herb seeds and plants, including some garden packages, with an emphasis on common culinary and medicinal herbs.

http://www.burpee.com/herbs

## Horizon Herbs

Horizon Herbs provides certified organic seeds, roots, and plants. They specialize in medicinal and magical herbs.

http://www.horizonherbs.com

## Mountain Rose Herbs

Mountain Rose Herbs specializes in seeds for medicinal herbs, either organically grown or sustainably harvested from the wild.

http://www.mountainroseherbs.com/seeds/seeds.php

## Nichols Garden Nursery

Nichols Garden Nursery carries herb plants and seeds, along with vegetables and other varieties. They practice "Safe Seeds" and sell no genetically modified or treated seeds.

https://www.nicholsgardennursery.com/store

## Nicky's Nursery

Nicky's Nursery provides herb seeds for culinary, dyeing, magical, medicinal, and ornamental purposes. They have a huge selection, including some very hard-to-find items.

http://www.nickys-nursery.co.uk/seeds/pages/herb-index.htm

## Sand Mountain Herbs

Sand Mountain Herbs offers native, medicinal, and Chinese

herb seeds and roots.
http://www.sandmountainherbs.com

## Seedman.com

Seedman.com carries seeds from around the world, including some medicinal and magical ones. Their site has some helpful lists, such as edible landscape, xeriscape, medicinal, and herbal plant seeds.
http://www.seedman.com

## Seeds of Change

Seeds of Change provides organically grown seeds, plants, bulbs, and tubers for various herbs and other garden plants. They have a specialty and medicinal section, too.
http://www.seedsofchange.com

## Thyme Garden Herb Company

The Thyme Garden Herb Company produces organic seeds and plants for various herbs, plus other herbal products and extra things such as mushroom spawn.
http://www.thymegarden.com

Starting in early spring, you can visit garden centers and nurseries to shop for seeds or live plants. Look in your phonebook to find them, or search online at http://www.gardens.com/local/garden-centers.

Shopping early means you'll catch the good stuff before it all sells out. Sometimes plants may get frostbitten and be placed on sale; you can usually find ones that will recover with a little care. Visiting a local nursery also gives you a chance to talk with the staff. They can advise you on which varieties grow best in your particular area.

Spanning winter and spring are the seed and plant swaps. Although some have a small entry fee, many of these are free, making an excellent opportunity for gardeners on a budget. It's easy to find culinary herbs this way, as well as some of the more popular medicinal or craft ones. However, some people are into collecting all kinds of unusual plants, including magical ones and unusual specialties such as dye plants, so you have a chance of finding just about anything.

Seed swaps usually work by posting a list of what you want and what you have, then shipping seed packets long distance. Many swaps are organized online, others in magazines or by gardening clubs. They may be direct exchanges between two people, or a jumble of one-way mailings among different active members.

Plant swaps are more often done in person, where everyone pots some extra plants and brings them to a central location to trade. You get to take home one plant for each plant that you bring.

Both of these swap methods promote herbs that are open-pollinated or can be propagated by division, rather than hybrids. Be aware that you may not always get exactly what you expect, though; sometimes people misidentify things. Swaps are also an excellent place to meet other gardeners, including magical gardeners if you're lucky.

### National Gardening Association Seed Swap

The National Gardening Association's seed swap is a free forum specializing in two-way exchanges of seeds.
http://www.garden.org/seedswap

### Garden Swap Shop

Garden Swap Shop offers a place to buy, sell, or trade plants and seeds.

http://gardenswapshop.co.uk

### Plantswap

Plantswap hosts forums where people can post want/have lists of seeds or plants.

http://www.plantswap.net

### Seed Savers Exchange

Seed Savers Exchange focuses on collecting and sharing rare and heritage seeds.

http://www.seedsavers.org

## Plants versus Seeds

Some types of herbs are available in only one form, usually because they are difficult to grow from seed. Saffron crocus, for instance, typically comes in corms, while asparagus comes as roots. Many varieties that come as seed are also available as plants. Rare or exotic herbs may be offered only as seed if the demand is not high enough for plants. If you have a choice between plants and seeds, pay attention to their respective advantages and disadvantages.

Seeds are cheaper to buy, and to ship if you are mail-ordering your herbs. They weigh less and take up less space. They are less prone to damage in shipping than plants. Selection is often much wider. You can plant your garden much earlier by sowing seeds indoors in late winter. Choose seeds for herbs that dislike being transplanted. This is also the best choice for covering large areas, such as naturalizing herbs for wildlife.

The main drawback of seeds is that they always take extra time to sprout and grow before you can enjoy your herbs. Also, young seedlings are quite vulnerable to pests, diseases, and harsh weather. Some herbs are difficult to sprout from seeds. More careful soil preparation is required if you are sowing the seeds directly in your garden, or growth medium if you are starting them indoors.

Plants give you a head start on growth, so you can enjoy your herbs sooner. If you buy them in person, you can pick out the healthiest ones: look for bushy herbs with no fading, spotting, or holes in the leaves and no roots poking out the bottom of the pot. Many herbs should have a strong scent, so you can check for that as well; usually the stronger the scent, the stronger the flavor. Well-started plants are more resistant to stress, especially if they have been hardened off properly to cope with spring weather.

The main drawback of plants is that they are more expensive than seeds. They cost more to ship if you are mail-ordering. Bigger plants also have higher prices than smaller plants. They can be damaged in shipping, or even just driving home from a nursery or plant swap if you aren't careful. Plants are also more prone than seeds to harbor pests or diseases that could be introduced into your garden.

In general, annuals and biennials are easier to grow from seed. So are some perennials that tend to be more leafy than woody. Herbs that have a wildflower or weed quality may also sprout very freely. Some good herbs to start from seed include amaranth, arugula, basil, catnip, chamomile, chervil, cilantro, dill, echinacea, fennel, mint, motherwort, mustard, parsley, peppers, sweet marjoram, and summer savory.

Conversely, perennials are often better to raise as transplants. They may not start as easily, but their root systems are more robust once they get going. Annuals that turn woody fast may also transplant well. Anything with a big root or bulb is usually easier to propagate from the ground up than by seed. Some good herbs to buy as plants include artemisia, chives, garlic, lavender, lovage, oregano, raspberry, rhubarb, rosemary, sage, thyme, wild strawberry, sweet woodruff, tarragon, winter savory, and wintergreen.

## Starting Seeds

If you're new to starting your own seeds, begin with a simple project. Choose just a few varieties of easy-to-grow herbs, such as catnip, echinacea, or parsley. Once you have more experience, you can grow more varieties and more challenging herbs. This also lets you expand your equipment gradually, rather than having to buy a lot of things at once.

Most garden stores carry supplies for starting seeds indoors. Some of these supplies are also useful for starting seeds outdoors. Necessary items include growth medium, fertilizer, containers, grow lights, and plant shelters. You can also shop for materials online. Here are some suppliers to consider.

**Burpee**
Burpee offers grow kits, growth medium, grow lights, heat mats, pots and trays, paper pot rollers, and other accessories. http://www.burpee.com/seed-starting

**Grow Organic**
Grow Organic sells soil-block makers, seed-starting trays, biodegradable pots, plant labels, heat mats, hand seeders,

transplanting tools, and many other supplies.
http://www.groworganic.com/growing-supplies/seed-starting
.html

### Harris Seeds

Harris Seeds carries light stands, heat mats, propagation trays, humidity domes, labels, watering gear, and more.
http://www.harrisseeds.com/storefront/c-30-seed-starting.aspx

### Home Harvest Garden Supply

Home Harvest provides nursery flats, rooting gels and supplies, row markers, seed sowers, growth media, heating equipment, misting systems, cloning and rooting systems, and plant health-care supplies. Look here if you're into home propagation beyond just seeds, such as cuttings.
http://homeharvest.com/propagationmain.htm

When planting seeds, first consider timing. If you plan to start more than a few seeds, establish a weekly planting schedule. Count backwards from the last frost date in your area. Seeds typically require four to twelve weeks of growth indoors before they can be transplanted outdoors; longer times may require transplanting to a larger pot before the garden. That timing varies by species (and care), so check the descriptions on the seeds you buy. You can also find some seed-starting schedules online, such as at http://herbgardens.about.com/od/indoorgardening/a/StartHerbSeed.htm.

Choose containers based on numbers and other concerns. If you're sprouting only a few herbs, individual pots—preferably biodegradable ones—maximize growth potential. Moderate numbers of seedlings benefit from pots or soil plugs gathered in a tray. Large numbers do best in specialized seedling trays with many small pockets. Another good option is to use solid flats full of growth medium, sow thickly, then thin the herbs before digging out the transplants. With herbs you can snip off the thinnings and use them in salad! Try to avoid plastic containers, or if you must use them, at least reuse them rather than throwing them away.

Use soilless growth medium rather than garden soil. For starting seeds, the medium needs to be very fine; a coarser medium is acceptable for transplanting tiny plugs into larger pots. Ingredients may include coir, compost, greensand, peat moss, perlite, protein meal, sand, sphagnum moss, trace minerals, vermiculite, and so on. Bear in mind that some of these are sustainable and others are not; if you're growing culinary, medicinal, or magical plants, you may want to be especially careful in choosing Earth-friendly materials. If you do a lot of seed starting, you may wish to mix your own growth medium.

Temperature affects germination and growth speed. Some herbs benefit from higher temperatures. Placing a heat mat under your propagation tray will boost the performance of your seeds. Take off about a week of growth time if you do this, to account for the faster rate. Note that soil temperature matters more than air temperature. About 75°F underground is good for many herbs, but check the individual species for exact details.

Light allows plants to grow and produce food for themselves. Indoors, herbs need supplemental light to grow. You can find grow lights in garden stores and sometimes also in supermarkets or hardware stores. Online garden suppliers also sell them. If you have more than a few herbs, a plant rack with lights is a good investment for compact storage and good lighting. Note that some species, especially wildflower herbs, may need light to germinate. Seedlings require twelve to fourteen hours of light per day.

Water is also necessary for germination and growth. The trick is to keep the growth medium damp but not soggy. If it's too dry, seeds won't germinate; too wet, and seeds or sprouts will rot. Seedling trays are often designed to soak up water as needed from a reservoir at the bottom. If you water from the top, you'll need a special mister to avoid damaging delicate seedlings. Use pure water, not tap water or softened water, which contains chemicals that may harm the plants.

Fertilizer provides nutrients for your herbs to thrive. An excellent choice is compost mixed into the growth medium, because you don't have to keep fussing with it. Otherwise you can use a liquid fertilizer, such as fish emulsion, or a compound chemical fertilizer. Begin fertilizing when seedlings develop their second set of true leaves, using a half-strength fertilizer about once a week. When seedlings are about a month old, use full-strength fertilizer according to package instructions. Remember to prepare your garden soil by adding compost or other necessary amendments before sowing seeds or transplanting seedlings.

## Transplanting

If you sow seeds directly in the garden, they won't need transplanting. If you sow in individual pots, they will need transplanting once, when they have several sets of true leaves but before they get spindly. If you sow in flat trays or in trays with tiny spaces, they'll need to be transplanted into larger individual containers and then into the garden. Pot them when they get their first set of true leaves.

Prepare the pots or garden soil to receive the transplants. Dig a hole for each seedling. Carefully lift the seedling out of its original container, or tear away the top half of a biodegradable pot. Place the seedling in the hole, making sure it sits at the same soil level. Fill and firm the soil around it. Water gently around the base.

Seedlings raised indoors should be "hardened off" prior to planting outdoors, so they can acclimate to the new conditions. First, lower the temperature and reduce the amount of watering indoors. It also helps to put a fan on low near the seedlings for an hour or so a day, simulating breezes and encouraging their stems to grow sturdier. Then put them outdoors for half a day at a time in the shade. After a few days, make it half a day in the sun. Then put them out all day in the sun. Do not leave seedlings out in the rain, wind, or very cold weather. The whole process should take about two weeks.

Finally, delicate seedlings may benefit from shelter in the garden. In full sun you may need to use shade cloth. In cool weather, cloches or row covers help hold in heat. Mesh tipis can provide shade and protect against wind or rain. You can usually discontinue the shelter once seedlings put out new leaves, indicating that their roots have sunk into the garden soil.

## Further Reading

*Burpee Seed Starter: A Guide to Growing Flower, Vegetable, and Herb Seeds Indoors and Outdoors* by Maureen Heffernan. John Wiley and Sons, 1997. Find out about starting herbs from seeds in your home or garden.

*The Herb Gardener: A Guide for All Seasons* by Susan McClure. Storey Publishing, 1996. Follow herb-gardening techniques through the year.

*Homegrown Herbs: A Complete Guide to Growing, Using, and Enjoying More Than 100 Herbs* by Rosemary Gladstar, Tammi Hartung, and Saxon Holt. Storey Publishing, 2011. Learn how to grow herbs and what you can do with them.

# Charming Morning Glories

### ⫘ by James Kambos ⫘

While growing up on my grandparents' Ohio farm, I was greeted by two things every summer morning: the sound of a rooster's crow, and the sight of Heavenly Blue morning glories blooming on a simple chicken wire trellis that covered one side of our front porch. My grandmother would sow the seeds in late spring, and by mid-summer they'd put on an extravagant show. Their intense blue flowers echoed the blue of the early morning summer sky.

I thought they were so pretty. I still do.

As a gardener you'll find this easy-to-grow annual vine to be the perfect backdrop for any herb or perennial garden. Morning glories come in such a wide variety of colors that I'm sure you'll have no trouble finding the perfect one to complement your color scheme.

And, as you'll see, the morning glory has a rich history. It not only was used as an ornamental, but was also highly prized by ancient magicians for its alleged mystical qualities. The seeds, and to a lesser degree the flowers and foliage, were used to communicate with the spirit realm and the gods.

## Botanical Information and History

Morning glories are a member of the Convolvulaceae family and the genus *Ipomoea*. The number of species within the genus *Ipomoea* is at least 500, and some experts say the number could be as high as 1,000.

Although the morning glory is a native of Mexico and Central America, it's believed the Chinese were the first to use the morning glory for medicinal purposes. They used the seeds in small doses as a laxative. By the ninth century the Japanese were growing the morning glory as an ornamental.

Native Americans also used the plant for medical reasons. They made teas from the roots for use as a laxative and a diuretic. They also dried the foliage to make a tea to treat headaches and indigestion.

Since all parts of the morning glory can be quite toxic, the plant is seldom used today by herbalists as a medical treatment.

It's the indigenous people of Mexico, however, who have had the highest regard for the morning glory as a sacred and magical plant since ancient times. Cultures such as the ancient Aztecs, Mazatecs, and Zapotecs believed, and still do believe, that the morning glory not only contains spirits, but that the plant has the ability to connect us with the spirit realm, and ultimately the gods.

The shamans of these ancient civilizations would drink a magical potion derived from ground morning glory seeds mixed with water to achieve a state of altered consciousness. Morning glory seeds contain certain types of lysergic acid derivatives, or LSA, which is related to LSD. Ingestion of the seeds caused powerful visions, which the shamans would use to communicate with the spirit realm. These visions would assist the shaman in discovering how to cure the ill, or help in enhancing their magical powers. The process usually involved grinding the seeds, wrapping them in a cloth, and soaking in water. Soon after consuming this sacred liquid, the shaman would begin a spiritual and visual quest to receive messages from the gods.

Today, consuming morning glory seeds isn't only illegal, it's also very dangerous. Side effects include cramps, nausea, miscarriage, permanent mental disorders, convulsions, stroke, and death. Also be aware that most seed companies now coat their seeds with a fungicide to prevent ingestion of the seeds. In other words, never attempt to use the seeds as a hallucinogen!

## Habitat and Cultivation

In Mexico and Central America, the morning glory is a perennial. In northern climates, however, it's grown as an annual.

Morning glories need some type of trellis or support and can reach heights of five to twelve feet. The vine is covered with large heart-shaped foliage. The lovely trumpet-shaped flowers are usually two and a half to four inches across. As the name suggests, the flowers open in the early morning, then curl and close in the heat of late morning or early afternoon. On cool, cloudy days, the flowers may stay open most of the day.

Colors include white, blue, purple, pink, and red. There are several varieties that are uniquely striped or are delicately edged in white. Each flower also features an attractive five-pointed star shape, which can be a contrasting color or can be the same color as the flower. The trumpets usually have a white throat tinged with yellow, but in some varieties the throat is pink. The *Ipomoea* moonflower is the only variety in the morning glory family that has flowers that open in the evening. The stunning, pure-white flowers are fragrant and measure about five inches across. Some gardeners plant them with morning glories so they'll have flowers blooming both morning and evening.

Morning glory seeds are easy to sow directly into the garden. Select a sunny or partially shaded location with average garden soil. After danger of frost has passed, turn the soil, then prepare the seeds. To hasten germination, nick the seeds with a knife or soak them in water for several hours. Plant the seeds ¼ to ½ inch deep; keep the seedbed moist. Once the seedlings appear (usually in seven to ten days), I usually stop watering, unless it's very dry—then I'll continue watering. When the seedlings are four to six inches high, you can thin or transplant them. Use a garden stake or some string to lead them to the support of your choice. If you plant by the "signs," morning glories benefit from being planted during the first or second phase of the moon, when the moon is in Virgo.

Once your morning glories are established, water them only during droughts. Too much water or a rainy summer will produce lush foliage, but few flowers. They don't require fertilization.

Apartment dwellers may grow these vigorous vines on a terrace. Simply sow the seeds in a large planter and thin to about three seedlings. Then place a small trellis into the planter and they should do fine.

## Favorite Morning Glory Varieties

No matter where you choose to grow morning glories—on a trellis, rambling over a porch, or climbing up a mailbox post—they are an old-time garden favorite that will always remind us of a gentler time. For many of us they conjure memories of summer mornings long ago. Morning glories are an inexpensive way to add beauty and charm to the garden from mid-summer to hard frost.

Here are the names and descriptions of a few classic varieties of morning glories that have stood the test of time.

### Blue Star
This variety is pale blue with a pink star. If you enjoy something different, this is the one for you. Grows to 6½ feet.

### Candy Pink
Vivid pink, this variety reminds me of cotton candy. Ultimate height is 10 feet.

### Carnival
This unique variety is a mix of flowers that have lovely pink and white, or violet and white, stripes on each flower. A compact grower; height is 5 to 6 feet.

## Celestial Mix

This morning glory variety is a mix of white, light blue, and dark blue flowers. Most have a contrasting star. Grows to 6 to 7 feet.

## Crimson Rambler

Red flowers with white throats make this old variety a favorite. I plant it frequently. A vigorous grower; height is 12 feet. Looks great covering a porch.

## Early Call

This variety is one of my favorites. It blooms a couple weeks earlier than most. It's sold as a mixture; the flowers will be pink, violet, red, and deep purple. Some flowers will be edged in white. It grows to at least 12 feet.

## Flying Saucers

Blue and white striped flowers make this morning glory a dramatic accent; interplant with a white variety for great impact. Height is about 10 feet.

## Grandpa Ott

One of the greatest morning glories of all time! An heirloom variety, its flowers are a little smaller than most, but they're an unusual color combination: purple with a red star. Vigorous plants grow to 15 feet and self-sow.

## Heavenly Blue

Introduced in 1931, this is the most popular morning glory. It has gorgeous blue flowers; height is 12 feet. A classic.

**Pearly Gates**
This strong grower is known for its white flowers set off with yellow throats. Looks great planted with red or blue varieties. Grows to 12 feet.

**Scarlett O'Hara**
This morning glory looks great rambling over an old, weathered fence. The flowers are scarlet with white throats. Height is 10 feet.

As I finish this article, it's a chilly, overcast autumn morning. But the Heavenly Blue and Crimson Rambler morning glories that cover my deck brighten this gray day. Gazing at them takes me back to my grandmother's porch. It's easy to understand why these old-fashioned vines have remained a gardener's favorite for generations.

## Seed Sources
Morning glory seeds are available at any garden center, or try these online sources:

Harris Seeds. http://harrisseeds.com.

Swallowtail Garden Seeds. http://www.swallowtailgarden seeds.com.

# Moon Shine:
# Herbs of the Night

### ❧ by Jill Henderson ❧

Often associated with the mystical, moon gardens have been lighting up the night for thousands of years. Adored by lovers and philosophers, these midnight gardens were places of secrecy and silence, contemplation and meditation, ritual and ceremony.

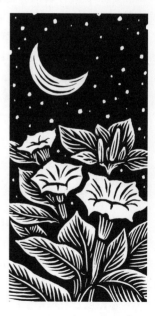

The moon has always given humankind a reason to look toward the heavens in search of answers and inspiration. The perfect time to relax and reflect is during the cool, solid stillness of night. The moon garden provides a place to do just that. It's no wonder moon gardens have become not only a popular gardening theme, but a true place of peace.

To our ancestors, the roundness and luminosity of the moon spoke primarily to the feminine form, and the moon became a goddess of fertility and bounty, a keeper of time, and the mother of all living things. Many cultures paid homage to the moon in the form of deities such as the Greek Selene and Artemis, the Roman Diana, the African Maou, and the Aztec Coyolxauhqui. Both beautiful and mysterious, the moon's soft femininity was countered by a vengeful power strong enough to push and pull the waters of Earth and the cycles of life. Those who worshipped the moon clearly understood this force quite well, performing traditional rituals and ceremonies to honor and appease her.

In ancient times moon gardens were not just for aristocrats, poets, and stargazers; they were places filled with valuable medicinal herbs used in the healing arts and religious rituals. Monks, shamans, doctors, and granny women have long been recognized for their contributions to the wealth of knowledge in the use of plants as medicines. Like many farmers of the day, these healers knew that seed should be sown in the light of a full moon and that root crops are best harvested under a waning moon when the energy of the plant is being drawn back down into the earth. This timing affects not only the plants, but also the potency and effectiveness of medicines made from them. With the moon playing such a critical role in the growing and harvesting of plants and herbs for food and medicine, it's no wonder moon gardens came to be not only functional places, but places of sanctuary.

Moon gardens are as old as the mythology surrounding the moon. Little is known about their true origins or when they were first intentionally cultivated. It was most likely a natural progression from an average daytime garden to one that included plants whose bright, reflective colors illuminated the darkness all around them, dispelling certain fears and scenting the night air. After all, what better place to meet friends or a lover than in a beautiful garden in the evening when the heat of a summer's day has slipped away? Like our early ancestors, we too have need of such spaces. Whether you want a special place to gather with friends or loved ones, or a retreat for quiet contemplation, the moon garden simply shines.

Growing your own slice of heaven need not be a complicated affair. Whether you decide to incorporate a few select moon garden plants into an existing flower or herb garden or create a full-scale masterpiece, only one thing really matters: that you make it a place you will enjoy.

If you are like me, the first thing you want to know is what kinds of herbs and flowers work best in a moon garden. Because they will be enjoyed primarily in the evening or after dark, plants for a moon garden have several things in common. To begin with, all moon garden plants tend to have blooms that either stay open all the time or bloom exclusively at night. These flowers generate the most "shine." White, yellow, and gold are all good color choices, though red and purple flowers can add a nice jolt of color for sunset viewing. Also, having one or two plants with sweetly fragrant flowers, such as night-blooming jasmine, white roses, or angel's trumpets, adds yet another layer of enchantment to the moon garden.

The second most important feature of moon garden plants is reflective foliage. In the next section you will find groups of flowering plants and herbs that have gray, silver, or variegated foliage. These plants add much needed depth and contrast to the moon garden by reflecting their ghostly forms. Many plants with gray-green foliage have the added bonus of being luxuriantly touchable and are sometimes quite fragrant as well. Artemisia and sage are two good examples.

The next group of plants anchors the garden by providing vertical lines and structural interest to the moon garden. These include ornamental grasses, small trees, slender shrubs, and even bamboo. Ornamental grasses have the added benefit of generating movement and sound. Last but not least, you can add a touch of functionality and whimsy to your moon garden by including a few white or almost-white vegetables, such as pumpkins, eggplant, tomatoes, okra, and peppers. Many of these vegetables are not only decorative, but edible as well. Imagine the ghostly forms of white bell pepper lanterns or magical glowing pumpkins in your moon garden. What a sight!

The following groups of plants are meant to get you started in your moon garden adventure. These plants are but a few of the thousands of wonderful possibilities. Use them as a stepping stone to find new and interesting cultivars to plant in your own moon garden. These lists include the plant's common name, the Latin name, and, where appropriate, the specific cultivar, as well as whether the plant is an annual or perennial. Please note that a few of the night-blooming plants are poisonous and have been marked as such. Use caution when growing these around small children.

# Moon Garden Plants

**Night Blooming**

Datura/White Moonflower *(Datura inoxia)* annual, poisonous

Cereus Cactus *(Cereus genus)* perennial

Night-Blooming Aroids *(Philodendron/Arum family)* varies

Angel's Trumpet *(Brugmansia arborea)* tender perennial

Night-Blooming Water Lily *(Nymphaea lotus var. 'Dentata Superba')* self-sowing annual

Flowering Tobacco *(Nicotiana sylvestris)* self-sowing annual, poisonous

**White and Yellow Flowers**

Cleome *(Cleome hassleriana)* self-sowing annual

Daylily *(Hemerocallis species)* perennial

Evening Primrose *(Oenothera species)* annual/perennial

Evening Primrose *(Oenothera speciosa var. 'Pink Petticoats')* perennial

Garden Thyme *(Thymus species)* perennial

Opium Poppy *(Papaver laciniatum var. 'Swansdown')* self-sowing annual

Oriental Poppy *(Papaver orientale var. 'Louvre')* self-sowing annual

Snow-on-the-Mountain *(Euphorbia marginata)* annual

Sulphur Cinquefoil *(Potentilla recta var. 'Warrenii')* perennial

Vervain *(Verbena officinalis)* perennial

White Four o'Clock *(Mirabilis jalapa)* annual

White-Flowered Borage *(Borago officinalis var. 'Alba')* self-sowing annual

Yarrow *(Achillea millefolium)* perennial

Yucca *(Yucca filamentosa)* perennial

## Gray, Silver, and Variegated Foliage

Artemisia *(Artemisia ludoviciana var. 'Silver King')* perennial

Coleus *(Solenostemon scutellarioides var. 'The Line')* annual

Common Garden Sage *(Salvia officinalis var. 'Berggarten')* perennial

Common Rue *(Ruta graveolens)* annual

Curry Plant *(Helichrysum italicum)* tender perennial

Eucalyptus Plant *(Eucalyptus gunnii var. 'Silver Drop')* tender perennial

Lamb's Ears *(Stachys byzantina)* perennial

Lavender *(Lavandula angustifolia)* perennial

Mullein *(Verbascum thapsus)* perennial

Munstead Lavender *(Lavandula angustifolia var. 'Munstead')* perennial

Red Everlasting *(Helichrysum sanguineum)* perennial

Sage/Salvia *(Salvia species)* perennial

Santolina *(Santolina chamaecyparissus)* perennial

Variegated Yucca *(Yucca filamentosa var. 'Variegata')* perennial

Woolly Lavender *(Lavandula lanata)* perennial

Woolly Thyme *(Thymus psuedolanginosus)* perennial

Woolly Lamb's Ear *(Stachys byzantina)* perennial

Wormwood *(Artemisia pontica)* perennial

Yarrow *(Achillea taygetea var. 'Moonshine')* perennial

## Vines with White Flowers

Clematis *(Clematis terniflora var. 'Sweet Autumn')* perennial

Moonflower Vine *(Ipomoea alba)* annual poisonous

Night-Blooming Jasmine *(Cestrum nocturnum)* perennial

White Cypress Vine *(Ipomoea quamoclit)* annual

## Ornamental Grass

Blue Fescue *(Festuca glauca)* perennial

Creeping Broad Leaf Sedge *(Carex siderosticha var. 'Lemon Zest')* perennial

Feather Reed Grass *(Calamagrostis x acutiflora var. 'Avalanche')* perennial

Feather Reed Grass *(Calamagrostis x acutiflora var. 'Karl Foerster')* perennial

Golden Hakonechloa Grass *(Hakonechloa macra var. 'Aureola')* perennial

Japanese Silver Grass *(Miscanthus sinensis var. 'Cabaret')* perennial

Japanese Silver Grass/Porcupine Grass *(Miscanthus sinensis var. 'Super Stripe')* perennial

Mt. Hakone Grass *(Hakonechloa macra)* perennial

## Trees, Shrubs, and Bamboo

Gardenia *(Gardenia jasminoides)* perennial

Ghost Bamboo *(Dendrocalamus minor var. 'Amoenus')* perennial

Harry Lauder's Walking Stick *(Corylus avellana var. 'Contorta')* perennial

White Climbing Rose *(Rosa species)* perennial

Yellow Stem Bamboo *(Phyllostachys aureosulcata var. 'Spectabilis')* perennial

## White Vegetables

Bell Pepper *('Bianca')*

Eggplant *('Alba')*

Eggplant *('White Egg')*

Eggplant *('White Lightning')*

Hot Pepper (*'Arrivivi Gusano'*)
Okra (*'White Velvet'*)
Pumpkin (*'Baby Boo'*)
Pumpkin (*'Lumina'*)
Tomato (*'Great White'*)
Tomato (*'Weissbehaarte'*)

Now that you have an idea of the types of plants that can be grown in a moon garden, let's get down to the bones! Start by selecting a location for your garden. It can be in a little-used corner of the yard for privacy or meditation, or it can sit smack dab in the middle of the yard. For trip-free nighttime strolls, be sure to allow plenty of room for pathways that are both wide and clear. If you are not the type of person who really wants to wander in the yard at night, consider placing the garden near a porch or deck where it can be enjoyed in relative comfort and safety.

Of course, your moon garden can be any shape or size you like, but the traditional moon garden shape is round. A circle can be arranged in many interesting ways. If the purpose of your moon garden is for relaxation or meditation, perhaps you might like to have a labyrinth of pathways within the circle that lead to a focal point in the center, such as a sitting area. A circle garden can be quartered to represent the four equinoxes, or wedged into twelve triangles to represent the months of the year. Half or crescent moon–shaped gardens lend themselves well to a fence or trellis against which climbing, night-blooming plants become the focal point.

Limited space or apartment living need not deter you from creating a small but beautiful moon garden. It's surprising how many plants can be grown on the smallest deck or patio using pots, urns, or tubs. Small wooden or plastic trellises are perfect for growing vining moonflowers or jasmine. To add some drama and flair to a small garden, use stands, blocks, or empty pots to stagger plants at different heights. Hanging baskets, window boxes, and many other space-saving planters are available to those with small spaces.

Water features are especially beautiful in moon gardens. Fountains make soothing gurgling sounds, while still ponds and birdbaths shimmer and shine with the moon's reflection. Particularly attractive in a moon garden are large structural elements such as glass orbs, statues, and sculptures. Objects that reflect light or make soft sounds are all welcome additions to the moon garden. Stones don't always shine, but they add a lot of architectural interest to any garden. Even light-colored pebbles in a pathway will glow in the moonlight, guiding you safely through the garden.

Obviously, a moon garden is meant to be viewed in the soft, ambient light of the moon, which isn't always available when we want it to be. For cloudy nights, or those of the new moon, a few strategically placed solar path lights will do wonders to make your garden shine. Even on full moon nights, one or two spotlights focused upwards or placed behind a predominant feature such as a fountain, statue, or trellis might just take your garden from pretty to stunning. No matter what shape, size, or configuration you choose for your moon garden, be sure to provide comfortable seating so you can sit back and enjoy the light of the silvery moon.

For thousands of years humankind has gazed into the heavens and been awed by the beauty of the moon. The ancient Hermetic teaching "As above, so below" is quite appropriate when contemplating a moon garden, for a moon garden is simply an earthly reflection of the heavens above. A moon garden teaches us to see things in a different light, both literally and figuratively. To see it correctly and to fully appreciate the smallest detail of a moon garden, we are forced to slow down and adjust our vision and perspective. Doing so allows a gentle light to really shine.

# A Gardener's Wildlife Habitat

### ☙ By Emyme ❧

My gardening life goes back twenty-five years. At times very alive and active, but for the most part quite dormant, my love of the earth and all its decorations resurfaced, and held, when I moved into my current home over six years ago.

During the first few years of caring for the yards and gardens, I concentrated on the flora. The care and repair of the house and grounds were so time-consuming, I barely noticed the fauna. They were just a nice distraction when resting after all of the mowing and trimming and planting and watering and weeding. Eventually the groundskeeping settled into a routine, and I discovered that equal to (and on occasion surpassing) the

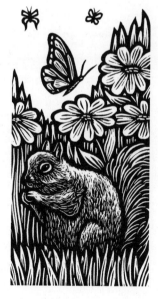

beauty of plants and flowers, one of the most rewarding aspects of owning and cultivating "a little bit of earth" is the wildlife. Rabbits abide, chipmunks amuse, squirrels annoy, insects alight, and the birds amaze.

More knowledge of those with whom I shared my out-of-doors was required. Once the pursuit of education began, three events confirmed I was on the right path:

- A visit to a birding specialty store provided seed, feeders, decorations, and more information than I knew what to do with, from knowledgeable and contagiously enthusiastic salespeople.

- Casual perusal of a colorful periodical uncovered previously unconsidered potential for decorating outdoor spaces: designs that use flowers and plants to attract birds.

- An inviting piece of junk mail introduced budget-friendly ideas in caring for the earth and her creatures, and optional financial contribution, regardless of where you live: city, suburbs, or country.

I suddenly saw the backyard with new eyes and determined to establish a wildlife habitat... only to discover I already had one. Should you choose to follow this path, it can be done with minimal effort and at reasonable cost. A cautionary note here: If manicured, leafless lawns and picture-perfect gardens are what you adore, you may wish to read no more. All but the most ecofriendly pesticides and weed killers are banned. Tolerance of disruption is to be expected when making homes for small mammals and offering food to birds.

Although there may be some who can manage to combine immaculate landscaping with wildlife habitats, for the most part they are at odds with one another. This has proven to be true for me, and it was quite a relief, actually. One of the previous owners of my home left a large dip in the backyard from a decorative pond. With thoughts of filling it inexpensively, I began a haphazard compost heap. Leaves, twigs, weeds, and grass...all are thrown in. Fruits and vegetables past their prime find their way there, as does the occasional out-of-date egg. Not very attractive to the human eye, the compost heap attracts all manner of bird and beast. Once in a while I used to cast a stray thought as to how it looked from my neighbor's second floor windows. Now, in the name of habitat, I can add to it without a care about aesthetics.

Other issues you may face:

- Chipmunks burrow, disturbing the lawn. Also, moles and voles create raised furrows.

- Rabbits build warrens in dense foliage and high grasses, requiring caution when trimming and mowing.

- Squirrels inconveniently drop twigs on the grounds and house while constructing their leafy nests.

But all of this is nothing compared to the satisfaction gained from creating a safe haven for these entertaining and necessary creatures.

And then there are the insects. Depending on the season, jeweled butterflies cautiously alight on the blooms of their eponymous bushes. Praying mantises in every phase of their life cycle crawl serenely among the plants. Dragonflies flit, fireflies glow, spiders weave, bees pollinate. Of course, there are mosquitoes and gnats. Some invisible something appears to chew on the rose bush. Nevertheless, nothing really attacks the plants; for the most part insects are left alone. Only rarely does something destructive come along and interference is compulsory—think mud wasps nesting on the brick façade by the front door and odorous house ants claiming the kitchen counter. I like to think I have been rewarded for good behavior in that I have never suffered any bite more serious than that of a mosquito. I have a plan in place to introduce the ever-helpful ladybug into this mix—maybe that will stop whatever is chewing on the roses.

Finally we come to what I consider the most excellent aspect of creating a wildlife habitat: the birds. Over the years the yard has managed to attract such a variety of them that I bought books and binoculars to aid in identification. At first it was merely the brown and black birds: mourning doves, sparrows, and crows were the only visitors. Perhaps an occasional robin or two. With the introduction of seed and feeders, the yard gained some color: bright blue jays, yellow goldfinches, and brilliant red cardinals stopped by.

Now, spring rains bring up the earthworms and robins nest by the front door—startling us and them whenever we exit. One year, house finches (sometimes mistaken for female cardinals) took up residence in the evergreens. Every summer the tap-tap of the woodpecker or northern flicker can be heard; they help with insect control and make fast and furious appearances—you have to be patient to see them. Starlings nest twice a year in the large birdhouse next to a rogue grape vine. Fall and winter bring the titmouse, chickadee, and nuthatch. As in any natural setting, the large feathered creatures and small furry critters collide. One hot summer day I witnessed a Cooper's hawk have its way with a rabbit. The carcass was left to me for disposal. Some years later, by the light of a half moon I saw what appeared to be a neighborhood cat take wing. In its talons, the great horned owl carried away another furry meal. The circle of life, indeed.

My yards and gardens are a haven for me and a habitat for wildlife. Even the least experienced gardener knows the seasons dictate the work schedule. Spring: clean up and repair the yard and gardens from the winter, plot and plan and plant. Summer: weed and prune in the cool of the morning, mow and trim in the heat of the day. Fall: bulbs in, annuals out, and leaves raked. Winter: resting, both the earth and I. Throughout all twelve months you can be sure of some or all of this: rabbits abide, chipmunks amuse, squirrels annoy, insects alight, and the birds amaze.

## References

National Wildlife Federation. http://www.nwf.org.
Wild Birds Unlimited. http://www.wbu.com.

# Rewilding and Reconnecting: Wildcrafting as Sacred Stewardship

### ☙ By Darcey Blue French ☙

There are many kinds of herbalists in the world: some who buy their medicines from others, some who grow their medicines in a home garden or on a farm, and some who wildcraft their medicines from the places where plants grow of their own accord. Many herbalists get their medicines in some combination of all these ways. I, myself, have for years used all of these methods for obtaining the medicines I use on a daily basis, and I want to share what I have discovered about the importance of wildcrafting our herbal medicines.

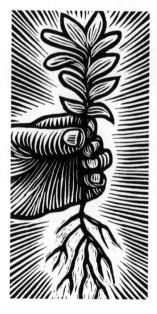

Wildcrafting plants is both a responsibility to and a relationship with the earth, the plants, and wild communities. Wildcrafting is a sacred act of reconnecting and rewilding our own spirits, and caretaking and honoring the earth upon which we live. It is a skill that is absolutely necessary to learn in our changing world and changing times, both for our own well-being and self-sufficiency and for the well-being, protection, and healing of our earth home.

Plants growing in the wild are subject to and influenced by the stresses of an unpampered life, with variable and often difficult growing conditions. Growing in the wild they develop higher concentrations of medicinal compounds, vitamins and minerals, and a stronger resilience and life force. It's no mystery to anyone that a tomato or a peach grown in a home garden and harvested freshly, at the peak of ripeness, is intensely more vibrant, delicious, and nourishing. Wild plants grow in soils undepleted by continuous cultivation, and increase their vital life force specifically because of the challenges through which they grow and survive.

By the same token, by relying on the wild plants that grow naturally around us, wherever we live, we are relieved of the need to provide extra resources to ensure a harvest. This is especially true in harsh, arid, or otherwise sensitive climates, where providing extra water or extended growing seasons with electric heating in a greenhouse may not be sustainable over the long term. Relying on locally available wild plants also has the benefit of reducing our impact on the earth. When we refrain from shipping medicinal herbs across the world, we save fossil fuels, promote ethical labor practices, and conserve plants threatened by commercial demand. While desired and valuable herbs don't always grow locally, it is important to remember that using what grows in your backyard and your bioregion is more sustainable over the long term. Using these nearby plants begins to put you into direct contact and relationship with the health of the land you live on.

## Sacred Relationship

Wildcrafting puts you in deep relationship with the plants you use for medicine. It connects you to the land you live and work on more than any other activity in the wild. Wildcrafting plants for food and medicine requires spending time in natural places focusing widely and deeply on the plants in front of you as well as the landscape and community around you. When you begin to wildcraft, first spend time sitting with the plant. Breathe deeply and begin to notice the details of the plant using your senses. What do the leaves feel like, how does the plant smell, and how many shades of colors can you see? Then use your senses to notice where the plant grows. Does it grow in the shade or the sun? Near water? Or on a dry hill? What other kinds of plants are around it? Are there many of the same kind of plant, or just a few? Do you see any signs of wildlife?

Always pay attention to feelings, memories, and sensations that come up when you are with the plants. Record your impressions, thoughts, and botanical notes in a plant journal that you can refer to year after year. This piece, the memory of plants, in place, is where relationship begins. Return, again and again, and ally yourself with that plant and that place. Use a field guide to identify the plant and make medicines with it, and take a small piece to wear in a medicine bag or to tuck into your pillow at night. You will begin to find yourself returning to the plant or the place as if to a beloved friend. These practices, when used every time you to go the wild places and plants, will instill in you a sense of the inherent value of the plant and the community it comes from. When your relationship goes deep like this, you will do everything you can to protect, preserve, and tend these plants and places. It is no longer a question of economic worth, but of love and care for something with value immeasurable.

## Respectful Sustainability

It is this care and urge to protect that which we love that make wildcrafting plants a sustainable choice for the long term. Ideally wildcrafting is done by the person who is actually using the plants, or a person who is serving the local community as an herbalist and/or teacher. There are instances where intense commercial wildcrafting of species like echinacea, goldenseal, and American ginseng has depleted and threatened the existence of these plants in the wild. Spending time on the land, in the plant communities, allows you to pay attention to the health of the land and the well-being of the species. You will notice if plant populations are increasing or decreasing. You will notice that in a dry year there are fewer plants, and take less. You will notice which plants also feed or shelter other creatures, and leave more than enough for all beings who use the plant.

When you wildcraft plants, learn proper harvesting techniques for each plant. Is it possible to clip a few leaves, or a runner root, rather than uprooting an entire plant? I use the rule of ⅓ when harvesting most plants (excluding very sensitive, rare, endemic, or slow-growing plants), which is: never take more than ⅓ of a single plant, and never more than ⅓ of a stand. Even ⅓ is too much in some cases. You will need to know your plants as individuals. Is it a slow-growing perennial root? Take less. Is it a vigorous seeder? Take more, but spread the seeds around. Does it grow only in this spot? Take less.

It is vitally important that we preserve these medicines for future generations. As the world around us is changing, we will need to become more self-reliant. These plant medicines are a gift from the earth for everyone. Our work preserving the land, the plants, and herbal knowledge are the ways we can demonstrate gratitude and be in service to the earth.

## The Practice of Crafting

Wildcrafting is a skill and an art. It requires a specific set of tools, knowledge, and attention to safety. Equip yourself with the proper tools so you can safely collect your plants and get them home and turned into medicine. Always travel with plant clippers or a knife. Many plants can be collected with your fingers alone, but tough roots, branches, or thorny plants will require a tool so you harm the plant as little as possible. You will want a good spade, shovel, or digging stick if you plan to dig roots. Digging roots in rocky soil by hand can be done, but it is a challenging lesson in preparedness. Always have a container to bring your harvest home in. I prefer baskets, canvas bags with handles, or paper bags. I never use plastic, as it can lead to mold or mildew, plus plastic bags degrade very easily in the sun and could possibly contaminate your harvest. Sometimes I'll even take out the glass jars and alcohol I intend to tincture my plants in, and put them up right there in the field for the freshest medicine possible!

Always remember to bring along all the tools you need to care for yourself as well, including:

- Enough hearty food and plenty of water
- Hat

- Sunscreen
- Journal
- Camera
- Bug repellent
- First aid kit
- Matches
- Rain gear
- Map
- Phone, or a specific plan to return left with someone at home

There have been more than a few times when I forgot just one of these seemingly minor details—and ended up shivering in rain on top of a mountain in a tank top, dehydrated and hungry and not paying attention to careful harvesting, or bringing home unexpected harvest in my hat. Part of this is the learning and adventure of wildcrafting, but just one unfortunate slip could be dangerous in some cases, so always be prepared to take care of yourself and anyone with you when you go out.

Here are some of the pitfalls and problems you should pay attention to and be aware of when wildcrafting plants. When I first started I was very wary of harvesting but also very excited, and fortunately had an excellent mentor to teach me where the safe, clean places to harvest were in my area.

You should take into account the cleanliness of the habitat you are picking from. Many lovely plants grow by the side of the road because of runoff and disturbed soils, but picking from the side of the road could mean the plants are contaminated by exhaust, oil, antifreeze, salt, or pesticides. Is your plant growing in an old farm field or an abandoned lot? Do you know the history of that land? Is it possible that the land was sprayed or subjected to other forms of contamination?

Know where you are collecting and the laws around collecting. Is it private land that you need to get permission from the owner to pick from? Is it public land that you need a permit for? It is almost always illegal to pick plants in national and state parks and in many other public and private preserves.

How comfortable are you in the place where you are picking? Do you feel safe, comfortable, and able to relax and pay attention to the plants and to what you are doing? Is it possible you may be interrupted by passersby? Are you prepared for that? Have you seen the plants growing in this area over time, or is it a new place for you? You may want to take less from an area that you are unfamiliar with in order to preserve the plant community over time. Take into account the potency of the plant: you can take less of very strong plants and still get good, strong medicine, and some plants tend to grow even fuller and stronger when they are harvested appropriately.

It is important to go to the plants with openness to what presents itself. Are you going out with expectations or specific intentions? You may go expecting to harvest one thing, and not find it, not get permission, or not find enough; but if you stay open, you may find someone else who wants to come home with you. Try not to go out with a sense of entitlement, but rather a sense of wonder and adventure. It is precisely these unexpected and unplanned connections that make up the bulk of our learning and connection with the wild.

Pay attention to *why* you are harvesting each plant. What are your intentions? Can that plant or that population sustain that sort of need? Have you asked the plant for permission?

Have you sat with the plant and expressed your intentions? Often the medicine most needed from a plant comes when we ask and come with a heartfelt intention. Make sure you give something back. It could be a drink of water, an offering of tobacco or other sacred offering, a scattering of the seeds, or making and keeping a promise to the plant ally.

I never take from the plants without offering something in return, and I often go to the plants to offer something without taking anything—songs, offerings, time, attention, and a promise to teach others about their value. This is the sacred relationship that, as herbalists and earth lovers, we cultivate carefully and attentively. One of my deepest, most sacred relationships with a plant is with an oak tree I have known for nine years. I have never harvested medicine from my friend. I regularly visit. I offer songs. I offer ceremony. I leave prayers.

Wildcrafting can be extremely rewarding when practiced with care, attention, love, and respect. One of the greatest rewards, beyond being able to spend countless hours of sacred time in the wild, beautiful world, is the sense of empowerment and self-reliance you develop as you work with the wild plants; and the knowledge that you know how to find, prepare, and use medicines and foods from the wild. You are no longer dependent on any other entity, institution, or organization to be able to care for yourself and your family. The earth is our home and our true provider of all we need—and being deeply connected to, in love with, and taking part in the reciprocal gifting cycle is one of the deepest healing and sacred journeys we can take. The plants are a sacred gateway into the wildness and magic present in all of life and our beautiful home, Earth. Step onto the path of a lifelong relationship with the magic and sacred gifts of the plants and the wild earth!

# The Gardening Wonders of Comfrey

### ⚹ by Charlie Rainbow Wolf ⚹

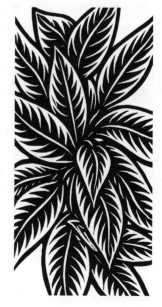

Comfrey has many healing properties and makes a valuable addition to the herb garden, but its overall use should not be overlooked by the serious vegetable or flower gardener. Comfrey has myriad uses, all of which are beneficial to anyone who is serious about composting, mulching, or attracting birds and butterflies into their plot.

The most popular strain of comfrey for domestic use is *Symphytum officianale*, more commonly referred to as Russian comfrey. It is a member of the borage family. The plant is perennial, dying down after the first frost and re-emerging with the first breath of spring. It is the root that is used in folk medicine, but we are going to focus on the other properties of this wonderful plant.

Comfrey is a very handsome addition to the garden, and it does not seem to be bothered by any garden pests or diseases. It has large ovate leaves that are dark green and covered in light fuzzy down. Some people find these little hairs quite irritating to their skin. The flower spikes consist of small mauve bell-like clusters, which gracefully bow down and sway in the breeze. Butterflies, hummingbirds, and other pollinators are drawn to the flowers, which have little to no scent, and the local bee population is also very thankful for these blooms in the garden.

Originally a European wildflower, *Symphytum officianale* is very hardy, and in some areas of the United States it is considered an invasive weed. It is wise to check with the local agriculture regulations before planting comfrey for a composting crop. It is tolerable of most climates, but because of the tuberous root it does prefer a moist location. It may not fare well in very salty or very dry locations. This plant won't thrive on chalky or rocky grounds either, for its roots need to go deep into the earth.

Once comfrey has been established in a growing location, leave it where it is. The most minute hair of root left behind will soon sport a new plant, as many amateur gardeners have found out to their chagrin! For this reason, comfrey is easily divided. The most popular way of propagating comfrey is simply to split a strong growing crown. It seems virtually indestructible.

The deep tap root is what makes comfrey such a wonderful garden compost plant. The root reaches down deep into the soil and draws up valuable nutrients into the wide leaves. When used as a mulch, the plant brings valuable potassium and nitrogen to the composting vegetation. The broad leaves of the comfrey can be laid directly around growing plants to slowly release their nutrients as they decompose.

Comfrey leaves and stems can be added to the compost heap to make a great green compost activator. Because they are so rich in nutrients, they not only add valuable elements to the compost pile, but they actually encourage it to heat up, thus speeding up the decomposition of other organic matter. Some people run the plants through a motorized chipper to break them up before adding them to the pile, but most who use comfrey regularly in their gardens agree this is not necessary.

Comfrey tea is another plant food option. The author has had great success making it using an old bathtub placed outside on cinder blocks. The harvested comfrey was wrapped in muslin and placed in the bathtub, and water was then added. The mixture needed to be stirred every day for about a week. The smell became more and more offensive as each day progressed, which was a good indication that decomposition was taking place! Once a nice black slime had been created, the plug of the bathtub was pulled and the tea drained into another container placed under the bathtub. The remaining slime in the muslin was added to the compost heap. Even the muslin cloth was reused, being placed under mulch to help prevent weeds near a vegetable bed.

Comfrey grows very fast, and one root system will soon give rise to a bushy plant that can grow up to a meter tall with an equal spread. Comfrey harvested in spring will rapidly reestablish itself for a second cutting approximately six weeks later, depending on its growing location. In a good year, it may be possible to get as many as four cuttings from the plants. For mulching and composting purposes, it is best harvested before the flowers form, but it does seem a shame not to let the wildlife feast on the beautiful blooms.

There are many reasons to devote a quiet corner of the garden to comfrey. The nutritional value for teas and composts, the instant mulch and plant food that can be created with the leaves, and the activity of the beneficial wildlife that the pretty flower spikes attract all make this an outstanding plant for the gardener. Aside from its gardening uses, it is medicinal and edible. Cherokee women used to smoke the leaves instead of tobacco. Comfrey also has a lesson to teach, for its tenacious manner and the way it keeps returning year after year remind the gardener that persistence is the key to success.

# Vanishing Herbs

## ᚙ by Carole Schwalm ᚙ

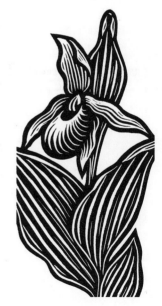

Rainforests like the Amazon and those in Madagascar are the "lungs of the planet." They are also home to potentially lifesaving drugs that are found nowhere else. The billions of acres are home to millions of species of plants, many that will be completely gone in forty years or sooner. One of these could someday save your life or a loved one's life.

We've tested only a mere five percent of these plant species, and many are anti-cancer drugs. How many potentially life-giving plants are lost in the hundreds of acres of rainforest that are burned and destroyed each year, about 1 to 1 ½ acres per second?

Saving the valuable rainforests filled with beneficial drugs sounds like a job for big pharmaceutical companies, or so you'd think! But, dear lover of the earth (that would be you), this is not the case. Oh, a few came, but they arrived in the form of "biopirates," and they stripped the forests and took seeds with them. The pillaging resulted in millions of dollars in profit. However, it wasn't adequate; the payoffs do not happen fast enough for pharmaceutical companies, for it takes time to study Mother Nature's complex compounds. Shamans, through extensive study, discovered that plants defend themselves against insects by manufacturing their own chemicals, which then became lifesaving knowledge.

The impatient pharmaceutical companies handed off to corporate co-biopirates. Large multinational companies swooped in and deforested to create land for grazing, timber, or corn and rice farming.

## The Shaman: A Living Treasure

A shaman is as valuable a resource as the rainforest plant life itself. He or she possesses limitless knowledge that encompasses thousands of years. Most shamans are seventy years old or more. When they die, their knowledge will die with them, unless the young study the old ways and unless the spirits call others to take their place.

Currently a group of international scientists are working in agreement with traditional healers and elders in light of drug research in the 107,500-acre tropical forest in Madagascar. Scientists are also working with native healers in Samoa, to glean, among other things, their generations of knowledge about bark, berries, leaves, and sap long used to heal coughs, malaria, and stomachaches.

# Herbs, Glorious Herbs

The Southeast Asian rainforest dwellers use 6,500 species of plants. The Northwest Amazonian rainforest dwellers use 1,300 species in healing. We cannot *not* mention some of the life-giving, lifesaving blessings of the rainforests and discoveries attributed to the Native Americans. They serve as reminders of what other wonders are there. They encompass coca, quinine, opium, and Taxol—a blockbuster drug from the bark of the Pacific yew. It is the strongest cancer drug on the market (one-half of all anti-cancer drugs are attributed to natural products).

In Panama, rainforest leaves and plant extracts are used to treat breast, lung, and nervous system diseases, plus the AIDS virus. They are also used to attack cancer cells and disease organisms that cause malaria and Chagas disease (the latter killing 50,000 people a year).

Centuries ago, Native Americans used natural herbs on themselves to treat conditions that settlers found fatal. The Hopi, Navajo, and Zuni used baby white aster for toothaches and rheumatism. The dandelion root is the medicinal part used as a tonic and a diuretic. The greens are a potent source of vitamin A.

Many of the wonders already found—like goldenseal, a natural antibacterial also used to treat asthma and colds—are disappearing because of demand. The lady's slipper, used for nervous disorders and female troubles, has been overharvested. Ginseng sells for $320 a pound because of the demand. How much more is unknown?

## Are You Inspired to Be a Shaman?

The spirits may call you: the urge to learn to be a shaman is a spirit message.

Do you have paranormal abilities? Have you cured by using your hands? Were you born with a caul? Have you survived a natural accident, an illness (called a "sacred illness"), possibly an illness doctors can't classify? Are you a coma survivor, or have you had a near-death experience? Are you a loner who enjoys going off in the woods to commune with nature, and you actually do feel at one with nature? Have you seen ghosts or a UFO? Do you often have unusual, vivid dreams? Have you experienced déjà vu? You can be part of the irreplaceable knowledge of the people.

In his book *The Medicine Wheel*, Sun Bear wrote: "The Medicine Man has eyes, ears, mind and heart open to see the magic that is always there." Do you see the magic? What you see can teach you. As the Medicine Men and Women discovered long ago, according to Sun Bear, the plants tell us which ones to eat to live well. One needs only to listen, just as we should pay attention to the valued treasures that are the shamans, the wise and indigenous people.

## References

Butler, Rhett A. Mongabay.com. *Rainforests*. http://rainforests.mongabay.com.

Sun Bear and Wabun. *The Medicine Wheel: Earth Astrology*. Englewood Cliffs, NJ: Prentice Hall, 1980.

# Bees, Butterflies, and Birds: How to Welcome Flying Friends into Your Garden

### ⤞ by Lisa Mc Sherry ⤝

After years of urban and apartment dwelling, I finally moved into a real house with a real backyard. I knew I wanted to create an environment that would attract birds, bees, and butterflies, and so the seeds of this article were planted.

Here in the Pacific Northwest (as in many parts of the country), blackberry and raspberry bushes abound—they'll easily take over your yard. Clearing them back or confining them to a designated section of fence can open up your yard and increase the amount of sun and space available to you. But don't get rid of them entirely! Birds love berries, and a small patch can keep a flock happy for days.

A key element to attracting wildlife is a reliable water source. My yard isn't big enough for a water feature such as a pond or waterfall, but I hung a birdbath in a shady, protected corner and make a point of changing the water every few days and refilling it daily during the summer. Most people have room for a birdbath, whether standing amidst a bed of wildflowers or hanging from a fence or porch.

Like many gardeners, I prefer to cultivate a mix of perennials and annuals, leaning more towards the plants that renew themselves naturally, thereby gradually decreasing the amount of time I have to spend putting in and taking out plants. Old-fashioned roses have a gorgeous scent and love to climb the fence, softening the lines that mark the boundaries of the yard. I particularly like Gallica roses, which are an Old World rose hybrid. They produce a long-lasting and spectacular show of pink, red, or purple flowers through the summer, with a heady fragrance. Bees love them. Another section of fence boasts a covering of clematis (*Clematis jackmanii*), which boasts large dark purple blooms that the butterflies and bees particularly love.

Lilies are easy to grow and propagate on their own, providing an ever-renewing and expanding collection of plants that honeybees love. Daylilies (*Hemerocallis*) are hardy and drought-tolerant and come in a variety of colors; a particular favorite in our household is the Stargazer lily (*Lilium stargazer*), which has an intense fragrance and blooms in mid to late summer. Most years we don't even bother to take the bulbs out of the ground, but leave them over winter and watch them bloom again the following year. A border that includes Queen Anne's lace (*Daucus carota*), lilies, echinacea (I especially like the purple ones, *Echinacea purpurea*), and sweet alyssum (*Lobularia maritima*) is a fragrant and pollen-filled welcome for bees and butterflies.

In a shady area, the stalwart hosta (*Hosta plantaginea* has a wonderful fragrance) grows beautifully along with Siberian iris (*Iris sibirica*), vinca (both *major* and *minor*), astilbe, azalea, and crocosmia (*Crocosmia aurea*). This garden will grow well and attract flying friends, expanding the possibilities of your garden.

Other plants the bees and butterflies love are some of the most common ones found in gardens: hydrangea, which produces flowers from early spring to late autumn; spring-blooming violets (*Viola*); rosemary (*severn sea* is a spreading cultivar with deep violet flowers); lilac (*Syringa*), which is used as a food plant by several species of butterflies; honeysuckle (*Lonicera*); and sweet-scented, night-blooming jasmine. Not as common, but my absolute favorite plant for bees and butterflies, is the gorgeous buddleja (often misspelled buddleia). Appropriately, its common name is butterfly bush and there are nearly a hundred species, the most popular of which produces white, pink, and purple flowers. Zebra longwing butterflies find buddleja flowers irresistible.

Slightly more exotic plants that feed the bees and butterflies include lamb's ears (*Stachys byzantina*); black-eyed Susans (*Rudbeckia*); the evocatively named love-in-a-mist (*Nigella*) and dragon's blood sedum (*Sedum spurium*); blue bugle (*Ajuga genevensis*); and smoke bush (Cotinus coggygria). If you don't have allergies, planting goldenrod (*Solidago*) will provide a bright spike of yellow, and bees make a spicy-tasting honey from it. Fleabane (*Erigeron philadelphicus*), a relative of the aster, does well in the Northeast, producing feathery pink or white flowers. Spiderwort (*Tradescantia*) is native to the United States, although more rarely found in the West and Northwest. Bee balm (*Monarda*) produces wildly varying flower colors ranging from crimson red to deep purple, and is also known as bergamot. Bright yellow coreopsis (Florida's state flower) blooms from June through August and leaves seeds for songbirds to enjoy during the winter.

Butterflies are attracted as much by bright colors as by taste, and they prefer yellow, purple, and pink flowers. Providing a broad variety of flowers will call them to your garden. Butterflies start appearing in your garden as soon as nectar is produced, which can be as early as March, depending on the climate. Feed these early visitors with spring-blooming shrubs, such as lilac, weigela, and witch hazel (*Hamamelis*).

Early spring is the most important time to feed birds, because the natural food supplies are at their lowest. Even if you don't stock bird feeders otherwise, this is a good time to do so with the seed the birds most prefer. (This will vary by species and habitat, so ask at your local garden center or use the oracle of Google.) Suspending feeders between trees increases the birds' protection from predators and keeps squirrels from eating all the seed. The rest of the year, birds will forage on insects, seeds, and fruit.

Flowers whose seeds are especially attractive to birds include aster, bluebell (*Campanula rotundifolia*), coneflowers (which include *echinacea*), dianthus, four o'clock (*Mirabilis jalapa*), gaillardia, delphinium or larkspur, sunflowers, marigolds, and zinnias.

Ground covers provide insect homes, a haven for earthworms, and a rich diet for hungry birds. Ivy (*Hedera*) and ferns

(*Pteridophyta*) are beautiful to look at and easy to care for, and help keep your hillside soil stable. Pachysandra is especially popular on the East Coast, tolerating cold winters and humid summers with ease. Bugleweed (*Ajuga*) shows bright blue flower spires in the spring, and vinca produces multiple waves of soft purple flowers that provide an early food source. I like mint (*Lamiaceae*), although it needs to be watched carefully so it doesn't take over the whole garden. Sweet woodruff (*Galium odoratum*), verbena, and thyme are other favorite ground covers.

Adding to your garden's perennial beauty, nectar-rich annuals attract butterflies and bees as soon as their flowers open. Zinnia (especially suited for the Northeast), cosmos (native to the Southwest), and Mexican sunflowers (*Tithonia*) are butterfly favorites. Marigolds, cosmos, and salvia are also food sources for a wide range of butterflies. Annuals keep your garden in continual bloom, providing color, fragrance, and an unending source of food for bees, butterflies, and birds. Keep clipping blooms as they fade to encourage new flowers, but late in the season just let the flowers dry to preserve their seeds for winter birds.

A garden setting that attracts birds, bees, and butterflies doesn't have to be purely ornamental. Black swallowtail caterpillars, for example, happily feast on the leaves of parsley, carrot, fennel, and dill. Other herbs you could include in your garden are yarrow, mint, chamomile, borage, chive, sweet basil, comfrey, and lavender.

I hope it goes without saying that avoiding the use of any chemical pesticides is strongly advised. Most garden problems can be solved with organic or natural solutions; a little research can provide a wealth of answers. Remember, too, that the caterpillars munching your leaves today are tomorrow's butterflies. If they are eating your cabbages down to the ground, try planting nasturtiums nearby to lure egg-laying butterflies away. Onions, thyme, or wormwood have strong scents that can keep caterpillars away from your edible plants.

Finally, I suggest that you research the plants native to your area and see how you can incorporate them into your landscape. Native plants are what will best attract the birds and butterflies in your area, as they are their original diet. Native species are best accustomed to the area's weather, soil type, and moisture levels. Once established, most native plants need very little coddling and often do well in areas where other species fail.

Planting a garden that attracts butterflies, bees, and birds is a simple way to create a wonderful place to spend time. Plan a viewing area and you'll have hours of entertainment year after year.

# A Gardener's Education

### ❧ by Emyme ❧

My gardening life began over twenty-five years ago. We lived up a hill from a small lake, and the water table was very high. The lawn was lush and emerald green all summer—no matter the lack of rain. In the front of the house I planted yellow daffodils and red tulips to greet visitors, a row of soldiers in regimental colors standing guard. In the backyard I planted annuals, and watched in amazement as the purple ageratum, pink impatiens, and white begonias went from sparse, two-inch babes to flowering beauties a full eight inches across. I thought I was great at this gardening stuff, but that

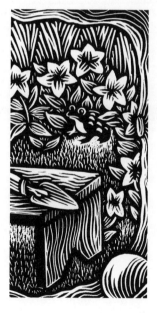

was all just the luck of location. Looking back, I had no idea what I was doing.

At the next house I planted annuals again: impatiens and begonias and dusty miller. Poor soil, no plant food, not enough water, and a crumbling marriage killed off that little garden. At one rental I planted marigolds and sunflowers. The outcome was an unattractive hodgepodge. It was seven years before I owned a home again, but the care and repair of the inside of the house left me no time or energy to devote to the outside. Another few years of apartment living and single parenthood put even the idea of gardening well on the back burner. In the winter of 2005, I moved into my current home: an American dream come true, a source of permanency and security. With apologies to writer Frances Hodgson Burnett, I finally obtained a "little bit of earth."

Similar to Burnett's *The Secret Garden*, the landscaping at my new home was a disaster. It would take far too long to describe all the changes I made over one very long, cold, and wet spring day three months after we moved in. I will say this: a previous owner had invested heavily in quartz stones and granite rocks. The rocks, arranged in a cairn-like heap by the garage, were moved to the backyard and currently mark the edges of three gardens. One oak tree and two bushes, an azalea and a rhododendron, also benefit from small, circular, granite-rock borders to hold in mulch. As for the stones, outside of a quarry I have sincerely never seen so many stones in my entire life. The removal and relocation of the stones is an ongoing project. Currently they are out of sight and off my mind. Their future status in the yard remains uncertain.

The first summer I carved out two little gardens in a shady corner. On one side grew a strange, neglected, little tree. Too much shade forced the tree to bend and twist as it sought the sun, with roots half out of the ground. It had to go, but instead of digging it out, the trunk was cut away to reveal a fascinating piece of natural sculpture. Around this stump I have planted and moved, replanted and removed, flora. After years I have hit upon an eye-pleasing configuration of textures and colors. Several heights of pink and lavender astilbe, the rich maroon of coral bell leaves, bright green sedum, delicate white lily of the valley, and purple balloon flowers—perennials all—take up the bulk of the eight-by-three-foot space. The companion garden is smaller and half-moon in shape. Sparsely planted, this bed holds only four plants: a small hydrangea in dusky blue and periwinkle, dwarf purple-bloomed butterfly bush, pink bleeding heart, and white astilbe. Where the first garden is a rough-and-tumble work in progress, the second is stately and static.

Nothing brand-new or perfect decorates my gardens. A child-size bench from a yard sale, antiqued white with hints of gold, is the non-flora focal point. Nearby sits a hunter green toad house from a garden center's as-is sale table. The plastic frog peeking out from under the balloon flowers surfaced while digging in another part of the yard. Resting within the twisted tree roots is a miniature, golden gazing ball rescued from a forgotten shelf in a nursery back room. Under the hydrangea sits a battered bee skep, and a hedgehog statue peeks out from the butterfly bush—both painted silver.

The only other planned garden in the backyard is circular, created in the mulch of a felled oak. It was haphazardly planted, with one large and one small green and white striped hosta at the north and south compass points, and a ground-hugging evergreen in the center. For years nothing did well there, and it never called to me, until I stumbled upon the idea of a green man. The large hosta at the top is "hair" and the smaller one a "goatee." On either side and slightly above the evergreen "nose," Mexican heather serves as lavender "eyes." Completing the face are pink geranium "cheeks" and a smiling "mouth" of red sage. Yes, imagination is needed, but I have found that to be so in every green man. These beds are my pride and my pleasure. Every year I add some annuals for variety—grasses or ground cover. Herbs and edible flowers are on the list for the future.

## Cuttings

Most of the plants and shrubs in my yard from previous owners had been severely neglected and were beyond saving. However, each year a tenacious, spindly azalea greens up, and orange-red daylilies provide glorious color. After much harsh pruning, the vine we suspected was grapes was left to grow, and bore fruit.

Due to weather and disease, we have been forced to remove some large trees. A few were oaks upwards of sixty feet tall and sixty years old. For every tree removed we planted another. Two flowering pears and a dogwood have been introduced, providing elegant off-white blossoms every spring. A rowan is planned; I look forward to the orange clustered berries.

I happily accepted lamb's ears and black-eyed Susans from a friend. The ears did very well. Too well. They were discarded after a few years when they threatened to override some other plants. The black-eyed Susans thrived and gave great pleasure until a well-meaning helper "weeded" them out. I mourned them greatly until the following year, when a few hardy survivors bloomed. They are being coaxed along, and that helper has been banished from that section of the yard.

One particular weed has presented itself as a great nuisance. Tropical soda apple is a ridiculously invasive plant with leaves mimicking those of the maple tree. Lured by tiny lavender and yellow flowers, and green and white striped, marble-sized fruit reminiscent of watermelon, the uninitiated will soon be cursing. For this lovely plant hides nasty needle-sharp thorns on almost every surface but the root. I have given up pulling them and now just mow them down. Their only salvation is they attract bees needed for propagation.

Every year something crops up that has been "naturally" planted. From bird droppings we have enjoyed random unfertilized maize—no ears, just stalk and tassel. Birds also "planted" sunflowers. The daylilies self-seed, as do the Rose of Sharon bushes. Recently, pumpkin vines grew from jack-o'-lanterns left to rot the previous fall/winter.

The front bed receives full sun for hours. One summer we planted marigolds of different sizes and all shades of orangey yellow. At the end of the season I collected and oven-dried thousands of petals for potpourri. A permanent part of this front bed is a rosebush, the flowers of which are a fine, rich shade of pink. No amount of pruning has harmed this bush,

# Planting Herbs

## ✒ by JD Hortwort ✒

Here's a conundrum for you: all herbs are plants, but not all plants are herbs. Here's an extension of that conundrum: all plants should be grown carefully, but not all herbs can be grown like common plants.

Regardless of where you garden in the world, most gardening advice starts out with this: *When planting, pick the right spot, then amend the soil with organic material at a rate of one part organic to two parts parent soil.* This works for beans and marigolds. It works for hostas and maple trees. It doesn't always work for herbs. It especially doesn't work when you are attempting to translocate an herb from a natural setting into your landscape.

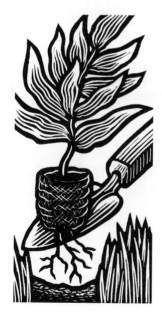

There are no two ways about it: Herbs are different creatures. They have different needs. They can be the most exasperating plants to grow and the most rewarding, if you succeed.

## So, What Makes an Herb an Herb?

Well, that opens another can of earthworms. Some people say an herb is any plant that is valued for its flavor, scent, or medicinal qualities. Emperor Charlemagne is alleged to have said in the eighth century that an herb is "the friend of physicians and the praise of cooks." Botanists will report an herb is the above-ground portion of a plant that does not become woody. So what are we to make of rosemary, which can mature to the point of having woody stems? Some experts say an herb is a plant that has no woody stems and dies back every winter. That pretty much leaves out plants like yerba mate and sassafras.

For the purposes of this article, we're going with the broadest definition: An herb is a plant, woody or nonwoody, perennial or annual, that is valued for its flavor, scent, or medicinal quality. To achieve that quality when we grow herbs, whichever of the three definitions we are talking about, we have to look at them differently than vegetables and ornamental plants.

Consider the desired result of a vegetable garden. Certainly you want tasty produce from your cucumbers or squash. But you want as much as you can get from these plants. The same is true of fruit trees, vines, and shrubs. These plants are high-performance athletes. Some last for only one season. Others, hopefully, will live for many seasons. Regardless, when they grow we want results. We want lots of tomatoes, bushels of apples, and pecks of blackberries.

So we treat the plants in a special manner. Like a goose destined to produce fois gras, we feed them extravagantly. We water them copiously. We monitor for insects and disease and treat accordingly. Yes, it's true that some gardeners take a natural approach to their production plants. They use organic fertilizers that create lower yields and are quite happy with that outcome. Still, even the amount of fertilizing done in organic gardening is more than the plant would likely get if it was growing in the wild (assuming it could survive in the wild). Plus, organic gardeners supplement with water. They take special steps to try to conserve that water—but they water, nonetheless.

Try this approach with herbs and you'll have compost within a few weeks. Herbs do not respond well to high fertilizing schedules. Only a few appreciate copious amounts of water. Most can take care of themselves very well, thank you, when it comes to insects and disease.

## A Different Tack

When growing herbs, we have to throw out our production schedules and take a different tack. Our herbs are meant to have intense flavors and/or scents that come from essential oils. These oils need to be concentrated. That means growing not a high-performance plant but a high-endurance plant. It means training a long-distance marathon runner, not a sprinter.

Herbs take conditions that would make a vegetable plant wither and turn that tribulation into a depth of character that we call essential oil. Feed them too much and the herb ends up sending a finite amount of essential oil into too much foliage. Overwater them and the herb will succumb to crown rot.

Interestingly, when you overfeed and overwater, if these two conditions don't kill the herb, they will weaken the plant to the point that it will become a mecca for insects and disease.

Starting with tips for growing the common kitchen herbs that many gardeners enjoy, begin by preparing a growing site. Of course, the planting site should be in an area that receives at least six hours of direct sunlight per day.

A sandy soil will require more organic material than a clay soil. Amend sandy soil with a bulky compost like aged sawdust. If this is not available, try soil conditioner. Soil conditioner is the remnants left after bark nuggets are packaged for sale. A good rule of thumb is to till the area to loosen up the soil. Next spread about one inch of soil conditioner over the sandy plot and till this in.

For clay soil, you need one part bulky organic amendment plus one part coarse builder's sand to get the right drainage. Use both sand and organic amendment. If you just mix sand into clay, you end up with brick. If you just use organic amendment, you might not get the drainage you need. The rule of thumb still applies: combine one inch of amendments over the area to be planted and till them in.

The next step is to check the pH of the soil. Most state land grant colleges offer soil testing services, although many charge for that service these days. Check with your local cooperative extension service to find out how to submit a soil sample. You can also purchase soil testing devices at most garden centers that will tell you the soil pH but not much more.

The pH is a measure of the acidity of a soil. The range runs from 0 to 14. Seven is neutral. Most U.S. soils are acidic.

As nature would have it, the greatest number of herbs need to grow in neutral soil. This includes culinary or kitchen herbs. A soil test will indicate how acidic your soil is and how to amend it. The usual recommendation is 50 pounds of agricultural lime per 1,000 square feet of gardening soil. If your gardening plans aren't so ambitious as to cover 1,000 square feet, then just factor it down. That's approximately 25 pounds per 500 square feet, or 12.5 pounds per 250 square feet, or 6 pounds per 125 square feet, or 3 pounds per 60 square feet.

If you have incorporated enough amendment into the growing area, you will likely find you can easily mound up the soil into a modified raised bed. No need to surround it with timbers or bricks unless you just want to. Creating a raised bed allows the soil to warm quickly at the beginning of the season and drain properly throughout the growing period.

Now you are ready to plant. Modern gardeners, being the impatient folks we are, like to purchase pre-grown sets. The advantage to sets, aside from the obvious, is that you know exactly what you are getting. But don't forego the savings of planting from seeds. Basil, coriander, dill, perilla, chives, hyssops, lemon balm, rue, chamomile, borage, and calendula can easily be grown from seeds. With plenty of patience, parsley, horehound, and sage can also be grown from seeds.

Certain other plants are better grown from sets or propagated from stem cuttings. They either grow entirely too slowly from seeds, or the offspring are unreliable in their characteristics. Mint is notorious for producing offspring from seeds that taste nothing like the parent plant. Others include valerian, oregano, marjoram, costmary, rosemary, tarragon, and thyme.

# Beyond the Classic Herb Garden

Most anyone can create an herb bed and purchase plants to grow there, but it takes special skill to encourage plants growing in one environment to accept a new location in your landscape.

When you decide to move plants from one spot to another, please consider taking a few precautions. First, desire does not supersede right. It's one thing to move a plant from the back of your property to the herb border, but it's quite another to take a plant from someone else's property without permission. In my area, some gardening groups will occasionally organize rescue missions if a property is being developed. This is especially true if there is a colony of rare plants on the site being developed. They always get permission from the developer first.

Second, make sure the plant you want to move is not on an endangered species list. Moving protected plants can get you in serious trouble if you are caught. Think twice about moving a plant from a different USDA growing zone. If you live in zone 7, for example, transplanting an herb from your cousin's property in zone 5 will be difficult. The growing conditions from winter through fall will likely be too different for the plant to survive. You can find your growing zone by doing an online search for the USDA zone map. (See the Research Help section at the end of this article.)

Properly identify the plant. Research it online. Talk to an expert at the local garden center. Check with a specialist at an agricultural college. If necessary, take a sample into the local cooperative extension office for identification. You may be surprised at what you learn.

As I was growing up in central North Carolina, my mother desperately wanted to move some clubmoss from the woods to a border near our house. Clubmoss has medicinal applications, but Mama wanted it for its fine, ferny foliage.

We tried countless times. We moved entire plants. We tried gathering spores and broadcasting them in the bed. We tried cuttings. Nothing worked. It was only years later that I learned clubmoss has a symbiotic relationship with a fungus in the soil. Without the fungus, no amount of coaxing will get clubmoss to grow in a new location. It's amazing how much you don't know about plants until you start researching.

Finally, make certain you understand what you are moving before you introduce it into the landscape. Herbs, whether medicinal or culinary, are wonderful things. But some don't belong in your landscape. Some plants are poisonous or, like pokeweed for example, have poisonous parts. You would not want them around little children or pets that might be harmed. Some plants are weedy. Witchgrass has an interesting seed head in the fall garden, but those seeds can take over a lawn. Japanese honeysuckle smells wonderful in late spring, but it's a prolific and aggressive self-seeder. Do some research before you allow "love at first sight" to wreck your landscape.

When you've done your research, it's time for work. Begin with your eyes, not your hands. Pay attention to the growing conditions of the plant you want to move. Many, many years ago as a novice gardener I coveted some mayapple I found growing at the edge of a dirt and gravel parking lot. *What could be easier?* I thought. *Here is a plant that grows in tough conditions. It should be easy to incorporate into the garden bed I just started.*

I'm glad it took some time before I could try to move the plant. Time taught me that the area where the mayapple was growing had a lot of organic material in the soil. It was growing in a low spot that tended to stay damp. If I had moved the mayapple into my heavy clay soil at the sunny corner of my house, it would have quickly died.

Observe the plant you want at different times of day. Just how much sun is it getting? Probe the soil to see what is going on below the surface. Once you understand the plant's growing demands, go back to your own landscape. Can you replicate the same growing conditions there? If not, leave your heart's desire where it is.

Your research should tell you whether the plant you are interested in is best grown from seed, from division, or from cuttings. Divisions should be done in either spring or fall. Cuttings are typically done in the spring or early summer after new growth begins. Seeds are obviously gathered from summer to fall, depending on the plant. For example, bellwort will set seed in mid-spring. Jewelweed makes seeds all summer. Pipsissewa makes seeds in the fall. Needless to say, if you intend to be moving a lot of plants around in the landscape, you are going to become very good at conducting research on the Internet.

If the growing conditions are right, prepare the area in your landscape before you dig the plant. Transplant shock has killed more plants than can be imagined. Get the plant up from its native area and back in the ground at your home as quickly as possible. Pay attention as you dig. How deep did the roots go? Did they run just under the ground surface or reach deeply into the soil? Remember to create the same type of space for the roots at the plant's new home.

Water well. If possible, create a temporary shelter for the transplant until it gets established to protect it from harsh sunlight or drying winds. An easy way to do this is to trim some light branches from an evergreen shrub and set them up around the transplant in a tipi fashion.

Monitor the transplant closely over the next few weeks. After roughly ten days, you should be able to remove the protective covering. After the first growing season (assuming the plant survives the winter), you can let your transplant grow without a lot of nursing. Herbs are such strong, self-sufficient plants once they get established.

After all, isn't that why we love herbs?

## Research Help

The Internet has become one of my favorite gardening tools. I often wonder what we did before it became available. Still, you need to be certain your resources are reliable. Here are a few to get you started.

Your local cooperative extension office can put you in touch with area plant experts near your town and at state land grant colleges. You can find your local office by visiting http://www.csrees.usda.gov/Extension.

The USDA Plant Database is a good place to start when researching plants growing in your neighborhood. This site will give you horticultural information, clues about where the plant will grow, and information on whether the plant is endangered or protected in your area. Visit the website at http://plants.usda.gov/java.

To see an up-to-date version of the plant hardiness zone map for your area, visit the U.S. National Arboretum website at http://www.usna.usda.gov/Hardzone/ushzmap.html.

Once you get started growing herbs, you may find your-self so enamoured, you have to know more. Start with the American Herbalists Guild for information on how to use herbs. You can read more at http://www.americanherbalists guild.com.

What we call herbs, some call weeds. So it should come as no surprise that a website on weeds would have good information on the look and growing requirements for some of the plants you have questions about in your landscape. Visit the Weed Science Society of America at http://wssa.net.

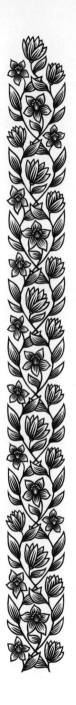

# Culinary
# Herbs

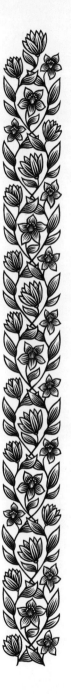

# Borage Bliss

### ✻ by Suzanne Ress ✻

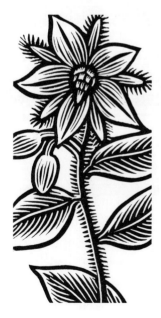

Early last March, after having done a goodly amount of research, I placed an order from an agricultural seed company for one kilo (2.2 pounds) of borage seed, which was delivered to me a few days later.

The previous year my three horses had overgrazed their favorite pasture, the one closest to the barn. I wanted to give the land a rest, as well as plant something that would be useful to us and also help renew the soil. I put a thick layer of rotted down manure all over the acre-and-a-half field, and soon afterward the field was plowed. I then hand-scattered the small hard black seeds over the entire field at the end of March, and hoped for the best.

One reason I had decided on borage was because I knew, from having a small plot of it in my herb garden, that bees love its flowers, and the pasture in question is located right in front of my apiary. Another reason I chose this particular herb was because its furry, rather thick and coarse green foliage, in such strange contrast to its delicate little blue star flowers, emits a lovely fresh cucumber scent when rubbed, and is delicious and very useful in the kitchen. And the third reason I chose borage over all other possible plant choices was that, as a "green" manure, it would add nitrogen and potassium to the soil.

For several weeks after sowing the seeds I watched and waited anxiously, worried that I had sown too early and the weather had turned too cold in the meantime, or that there was too much rain, or not enough rain, or that the crows would eat all the seeds before they sprouted.

I needn't have worried! By mid-June the pasture was crowded with the strangely beautiful hairy stalked plants, their tender leaves as large as pineapples, their more slender furry red peduncles sporting hundreds of thousands of sky blue, violet blue, and pinkish violet star-shaped blossoms. Above all of this was a happily humming golden veil of honeybees.

Borage gets its Latin name, *Borago officinalis*, from the Benedictine monks who grew it in medicinal herb gardens for use in their apothecaries, hence its species name, *Officinalis*, conferred only on herbs of prime medicinal value. Borage's family name, Boraginaceae, is based on its most prominent genus, borage! In fact, the family of Boraginaceae has only two or three other known members. The root of its name most likely comes from an old French or Italian word meaning "hairy."

Borage is also commonly known as Starflower, Beebread, or Herb of Gladness. Its sprightly blue flowers have five petals and look exactly like little blue stars. The flowers can range in color from brightest blue, to blue violet, to pink, but there is also a cultivar that produces only white flowers. It is rumored that a blue dye can be obtained from the flowers by macerating them for several days in alcohol. However, the blue color in the alcohol will change to pink if it comes in contact with anything even slightly acidic.

Each borage blossom is held by a slender red peduncle with stiff white hairs, and has five darker blue or violet protruding stamens, with black or very dark blue anthers. The flowers produce four "nutlets," or hard black hulled seeds. The fine white hairs that cover the plant's leaves and stems are stiff, like cactus hairs, and look as if they would prick, but they don't! Just looking at a borage plant in bloom can make your heart glad, for it appears both rustic and elegant, and earthy and magical, at the same time.

Borage's fresh cucumber scent is due to the same natural chemical process that produces the odor in cucumbers, as the plant's linoleic acid cleaves to its C9 carbonyls.

Borage loves full sun and is not very picky about its soil quality. Although it is not considered a plant for extremely dry conditions, it can get along fine for quite some time without water. It is an annual, but left to its own devices will self-seed, reappearing in your garden year after year.

Once the plant has finished blooming and produced its seeds, it will wither and dry up, becoming a gray corpse of its former self. If you burn these dried plants, they pop and sparkle due to the high percentage of mineral salts they contain.

One of borage's folk names, Herb of Gladness, comes from the belief that drinking a wine punch in which borage flowers have been macerated produces both gladness and courage in she who imbibes. Only in recent years have medical scientists at least partially discovered why this is true.

## Culinary Uses

Borage greens are very high in minerals. A 100 gram (3.5 ounce) serving of raw borage contains 9% of the recommended daily adult requirement of calcium, 18% of the recommended iron, 10% of the potassium, 13% of the magnesium, and 17% of the manganese. With only 21 calories to a serving, and 84% of the Recommended Daily Allowance of vitamin A, these greens truly pack a punch! The raw greens can be chopped up and added to mixed salads. They have a fresh cucumber-like taste, but because of their hairiness, unless they are very finely chopped or processed, some people find them texturally unpleasant to eat.

Here is an old German recipe for an interesting green sauce that contains raw borage.

*German Grune Sosse*

Process 2 hard-boiled egg yolks with 2 ounces fresh borage leaves, 2 ounces parsley, 2 ounces watercress, 1 ounce chervil, 1 ounce sorrel, 1 ounce chives, and 1 ounce salad burnet. Trickle 1 tablespoon olive or walnut oil into the food processor while it is still running. Then turn off the processor, put the green mixture into a bowl, and stir in 1 ½ cups of sour cream or plain Greek yogurt. Add a little salt, pepper, and a few drops of vinegar, and stir well. This uncooked sauce is commonly served over potatoes, beef, or fish.

Personally, I prefer my borage cooked. The hairiness of the leaves disappears entirely, and the leaves can be used in any of the same ways as spinach. Try borage in risotto, or as a stuffing for vegetables or rolled meat or fish. It can be used in baked pasta dishes with cheese, in quiche or other savory pies, in omelets, in soufflés, in soups, or as a steamed vegetable side dish simply dressed with olive oil.

One of my favorite ways to serve and eat borage is in a simple creamed soup.

### Cream of Borage Soup

Pour about an inch of water into a large pot and bring it to a simmer, then put in as many borage leaves as will fit. Steam them, stirring up the ones from the bottom occasionally, until all are wilted.

In another, soup-sized pot, melt 2–3 tablespoons of butter. Stir in 2–3 tablespoons flour, then press the wilted borage in the other pot with a slotted spoon, and add all the resulting liquid, stirring constantly. Add a quart of good-quality vegetable broth, stirring all the while. When it begins to thicken and simmer, turn off the flame for a moment and finely chop the previously cooked borage greens. Add these to the soup, stir well, then add one cup of crème fraiche, sour cream, or plain unsweetened Greek yogurt. Stir again, then heat for a few moments but do not boil. Serve with plenty of grated Parmigiano and freshly grated black pepper.

Borage's pretty blue flowers can also be used in culinary creations. I love putting them on top of a green salad. They look magical, and add a fresh cucumber taste. They can also be candied and used to decorate cakes, cupcakes, puddings, or other desserts. They can be frozen into ice cubes and used in fancy drinks and punches. Traditionally the British Pimm's Cup cocktail is served with a few fresh borage flowers floating on top. This is certainly a carryover from the ancient borage-wine punch.

*Borage Wine Punch*
Blend 1 bottle of good dry white wine with ½ cup fine brandy and 2 tablespoons mild (preferably borage) honey, until the honey dissolves completely. Add the juice from half a lemon and ⅓ to ½ cup fresh blue borage flowers. Stir well and chill for 1–3 hours. Just before serving, add 1 bottle chilled sparkling white wine or champagne.

## Medicinal Uses and Health Benefits
The oil that comes from borage seeds contains the highest known plant source of gamma-linolenic acid (GLA), about twice the amount found in evening primrose oil. GLA is an omega-6 fatty acid, and borage seeds contain 20% GLA. Borage seeds also contain about 35% linoleic acid, which cannot be manufactured by the human body but must be taken in as food or supplements. It is necessary for the proper functioning of the brain and metabolism, and for the healthy growth of hair, skin, and nails.

GLA is known to improve mood by reducing stress, and is prescribed to reduce the hot flash symptoms of menopause, for relief of premenstrual tension, migraine, mild depression, and irritability. Perhaps this is one of the reasons the ancients called borage the Herb of Gladness. GLA has been shown to help reduce both systolic and diastolic blood pressure in hypertensive patients, as in olden times, when borage seeds were given to cure heart disease. It has also been used effectively to control allergic reactions in affected people, and as a supplement to increase bone density in those at risk for osteoporosis.

Research is ongoing concerning GLA's role in reducing symptoms of eczema, Attention Deficit Disorder and hyperactivity, rheumatoid arthritis, and as a booster in breast cancer treatments.

Borage greens and roots were and still are used medicinally for their diuretic, demulcent, and emollient properties in the treatment of such ailments as diarrhea, bronchitis, and sore, reddened eyes. A poultice can be made of fresh borage leaves and applied to inflamed or swollen parts of the body (or closed eyes) as an effective anti-inflammatory.

Borage leaves can also be used to make a refreshing face pack for dry-skin types.

### Borage Face Pack

Pour 1 cup boiling water over 1 cup chopped fresh borage leaves and leave to cool to room temperature. In the meantime, beat 1 egg yolk with 1 teaspoon fresh yeast, 2 teaspoons almond oil, and a little warm water, to make a paste. Add 1 tablespoon of the borage-infused liquid, mix well, and spread all over your face. Then lie back and relax for 10–15 minutes, and daydream of flying over a field of blooming blue borage flowers. Rinse your face with warm, preferably softened, water, and generously apply moisturizer while your face is still damp.

## Honey Flow and Green Manure

Although borage is an excellent choice as both a honey-producing plant and a green manure, it cannot do both jobs simultaneously to the best of its ability!

A green manure is any crop or ground-covering plant usually grown on depleted soil that needs improving. Borage is considered a good green manure because it fixes nitrogen and adds potassium to the soil. It also has a long tap root that brings nutrients up from the deeper layers of soil to its leaves. In order for all these nutrients to be added back into the soil's upper layer, the green plants must be cut down, chopped up, and plowed back into the soil. This should preferably be done before, or immediately after, the plants flower. If they are left to flower too long, the first flowers will go to seed and you will be growing borage again the following year.

As for honey production, naturally the only part of borage that interests bees is the flowers. Since borage blooms continuously for several weeks and then quickly withers and dies, it is extremely difficult, maybe impossible, to cut it down while it is still green and finished flowering, but before any of the flowers have gone to seed. I think that in order to use it most effectively as a green manure, one would have to forget about using it for a honey flow, and vice versa.

Because of the weather conditions and the precocious blooming time of the other main local honey plants in my area this year, the bees had very little forage at the time their hive populations were highest, when the borage was in bloom. So I allowed the borage to finish flowering and die down naturally.

Although it is less effective as a green manure to allow the plants to die before plowing them back into the earth, this does still add nutrients and immediately increases biomass in the soil, which brings in more beneficial microorganisms. The activity of decomposition (think of your compost heap) increases the soil's aeration and ability to retain water. Used as a smaller-scale green manure—for example, in overused vegetable or annual herb plots—borage is an excellent choice.

Since the discovery, only some years ago, that borage's seeds are a major producer of GLA, it has become a profitable farm crop. For this reason, borage flowers are now one of Britain's main honey sources. The nectar produces a white or very pale golden honey, naturally higher in sucrose than many other honeys, and hence especially sweet. Its flavor is prized as delicate and mildly floral.

## Borage in Art

In sixteenth- and seventeenth-century Elizabethan England, borage flowers were a favorite embroidery emblem, symbolizing courage and gladness of heart. Certainly because of their symbolism, but also probably because they make such a simple and pretty motif, borage flowers were embroidered on ladies' fancy jackets and bodices, gentlemen's nightcaps, robes, and gloves, as well as on pillow covers, cloth book bindings, flags, banners, and more. The flowers were also frequently used as motifs in family crests and in medieval heraldry and coats of arms.

In the secret language of flowers, invented and popularized in the early 1800s and used for symbolic communication usually between lovers to send coded messages, oddly enough borage flowers meant "your attentions are not welcome"!

Throughout its long and illustrious history, the borage plant's greens and flowers have always played a very important role in many facets of human life. I find it amazing that we still do not know all this plant is capable of doing for us.

# The Gift of Spice

### ❧ by Jill Henderson ❧

Since the dawn of time humans have gathered and used wild plants for food and medicine. As their collective knowledge grew, they began to prepare and use them in new and creative ways. From simple seasonings to food preservatives, and from ritual offerings to healing medicines, herbs and spices have touched the lives of humankind for hundreds of thousands of years.

We often associate spices with hard, dry bits of ground-up plant material. But a spice can be made from almost any portion of a plant in any form, including leaves, twigs, seed pods, bulbs, and rhizomes. The famous Balm of Gilead is a sap resin gathered from the emerging leaf buds

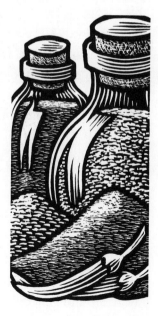

of the common balsam poplar. Some spices, such as garlic and ginger, are used both fresh and dry. Even flowers and parts of flowers are used as spices. The delicate and luxuriantly expensive spice saffron is the dried, thread-like stigmas of the saffron crocus, which are picked by hand.

Whether humans first used spices as food, preservative, or medicine is unknown. The only thing that is certain is that they loved them. In fact, the desire for new and unusual spices drove exploration for the better part of 5,000 years. It spawned wars and rivalries, built empires and kingdoms, and made men rich beyond their dreams. Had Christopher Columbus not been searching for a new, faster trade route to the Spice Islands, America might not have been colonized for another 500 years.

Spices have also played a role in the quest for spiritual knowledge, the development of medicine, the refinement of scientific formulation, and the timeless pursuit of everlasting life. As far back as modern archeology can take us, humans have used spices to express love, appease or thank the gods, anoint the dead, and garner favor among the living. Rarity and expense made a gift of spice one of the highest forms of respect.

Indeed, spices were among the world's most valuable commodities. For thousands of years the cost and rarity of spice was comparable to that of gold or diamonds. Only fifty years ago it would have been highly unusual to find a local source of the spices needed to create the kinds of international cuisine we crave today. In our modern society, we take for granted the availability, reasonable cost, and wide variety of spices on grocery store shelves.

The general availability and the reasonable price of spice today do not make it any less precious, because, though widely available and generally affordable, spices still aren't cheap. It might surprise you to learn how many people have never indulged in the heady flavors of high-quality, freshly prepared spice blends. This is what makes a gift of spice just as valuable and highly regarded today as it was a thousand years ago.

The following are ten of the most widely used spice blends, which have been customized to suit a variety of culinary tastes. Each recipe was formulated using the most common forms of spices available and can be prepared using either the small or large batch recipe (amounts for large batch recipes are in parentheses). If using whole, fresh, or otherwise unprocessed ingredients, you may need to grind them to the desired consistency. A coffee grinder used just for spices works exceptionally well. To make any of these spice blends, simply place all the ingredients in a large covered vessel, shake, and seal. If you like to play with your food, adding a bit more of one ingredient or substituting another will add your personal touch to a wonderful gift of spice.

# The Recipes

*Fabulous All Season Salt*

¾ cup salt (1 ½ cups)

¼ cup paprika (½ cup)

1 ½ tablespoons garlic powder (2 tablespoons)

1 ½ teaspoons black pepper (1 tablespoon)

1 ½ teaspoons white pepper (1 tablespoon)

1 ½ teaspoons thyme (1 tablespoon)

1 ½ teaspoons marjoram (1 tablespoon)

1 teaspoon onion powder (2 teaspoons)

1 teaspoon ground celery seed (2 teaspoons)

Salty spicy goodness in a jar! This spice blend is excellent on just about anything you can imagine. Try it on creamy chicken, fish or tuna salad, roasted vegetables, poultry, fish, beef, pork...the sky's the limit!

*Yield:* About 2 ⅓ and 4 cups.

### Bella Italian Seasoning

⅔ cup oregano (1 ⅓ cups)

⅔ cup basil (1 ⅓ cups)

¼ cup thyme (½ cup)

¼ cup marjoram (½ cup)

2 tablespoons rosemary (¼ cup)

1 tablespoon garlic powder (2 tablespoons)

2 teaspoons onion powder (4 teaspoons)

1 teaspoon red pepper (2 teaspoons)

1 teaspoon black pepper (2 teaspoons)

*Bella* means "beautiful" in Italian, and this spice blend makes any Italian dish stand out from the crowd. Don't forget to try it on roasted potatoes or tomatoes for a taste-tempting treat!

*Yield:* About 2 and 4 cups.

### Tex-Mex Power Blend

¼ cup ground red chilies (½ cup)

2 tablespoons ground coriander (¼ cup)

2 tablespoons salt (¼ cup)

2 tablespoons oregano (¼ cup)

2 tablespoons cumin (¼ cup)

1 tablespoon garlic powder (2 tablespoons)

1 tablespoon onion powder (2 tablespoons)

1 tablespoon paprika (2 tablespoons)

2 ¼ teaspoons black pepper (1 ½ tablespoons)

2 ¼ teaspoons sugar (1 ½ tablespoons)

1 teaspoon cayenne (2 teaspoons)

The level of heat in this spice blend depends on the kind of chilies you use. Perfect for Tex-Mex tacos, chili, burritos, beans, chicken, and beef. Makes an excellent fajita grill rub.

*Yield:* About 2 and 4 cups.

### Fish & Seafood Rub

½ cup sea salt (1 cup)

½ cup garlic powder (1 cup)

¼ cup dried marjoram (½ cup)

¼ cup dried thyme (½ cup)

¼ cup savory (½ cup)

¼ cup garlic powder (½ cup)

3 tablespoons onion powder (6 tablespoons)

2 tablespoons black pepper (¼ cup)

2 tablespoons white pepper (¼ cup)

1 tablespoon cayenne pepper (2 tablespoons)

1 tablespoon fennel seed (2 tablespoon)

2 teaspoons sweet paprika (4 teaspoons)

2 teaspoons dry lemon zest (4 teaspoons)

1 teaspoon ground bay leaf (2 teaspoons)

Use as a rub when grilling, baking, or pan-searing fish and shrimp. Add a tablespoon of rub to 1 cup of flour for deep frying. Blend into oil, mayonnaise, or melted butter to make a delectable seafood dip or sauce.

*Yield:* About 2 ½ and 5 cups.

### Grill-All Barbeque Seasoning

1 cup chili powder (2 cups)

½ cup salt (1 cup)

6 tablespoons onion powder (⅓ cup)

4 teaspoons cumin (2 ½ tablespoons)

4 teaspoons garlic powder (2 ½ tablespoons)

2 teaspoons paprika (1 tablespoon)

2 teaspoons brown sugar (1 tablespoon)

2 teaspoons cayenne (1 tablespoon)

2 teaspoons hickory flavoring (1 tablespoon)

1 teaspoon black pepper (2 teaspoons)

1 teaspoon dry mustard (2 teaspoons)

1 teaspoon dry ground lemon zest (2 teaspoons)

1 teaspoon nutmeg (2 teaspoons)

When you want to grill, this is your go-to seasoning blend. It has the perfect blend of sweet and hot to really bring out the flavor of meat, chicken, and vegetables.

*Yield:* About 2 ¼ and 4 cups.

### Holiday Pie & Bread Spice Blend

¾ cup ground cinnamon (1 ½ cups)

½ cup dry ground orange peel (1 cup)

¼ cup ground anise seed (½ cup)

¼ cup ground fennel seed (½ cup)

¼ cup ground ginger (½ cup)

2 tablespoons ground cardamom (¼ cup)

2 tablespoons ground nutmeg (¼ cup)

4 teaspoons ground cloves (2 ½ tablespoons)

Don't wait for the holidays to create wonderfully rich breads, pies, cakes, muffins, cookies, cider, fruit compote, and eggnog. *Yield:* About 2 ½ cups to 5 cups.

*New Orleans Cajun-Style Spice Blend*

¼ cup red bell pepper flakes (½ cup)

¼ cup parsley flakes (½ cup)

3 tablespoons onion powder (⅓ cup)

3 tablespoons garlic powder (⅓ cup)

2 tablespoons black pepper (¼ cup)

2 tablespoons white pepper (¼ cup)

2 tablespoons paprika (¼ cup)

2 tablespoons cumin (¼ cup)

1 tablespoon ground bay leaf (2 tablespoons)

1 tablespoon celery seed (2 tablespoons)

1 tablespoon ground mustard seed (2 tablespoons)

1 ½ teaspoons thyme (3 teaspoons)

1 ½ teaspoons oregano (3 teaspoons)

1 ½ teaspoons cayenne (3 teaspoons)

1 ½ teaspoons basil (3 teaspoons)

This superb spice blend makes fantastic gumbo and a tasty rub and marinade for roasting or grilling beef, pork, or chicken. *Yield:* About 2 ¼ and 5 ½ cups.

*Salt-Free Sensation*

¼ cup garlic powder (½ cup)

¼ cup onion powder (½ cup)

3 tablespoons savory (⅓ cup)

3 tablespoons powdered lemon zest (⅓ cup)

3 tablespoons dried basil (⅓ cup)

3 tablespoons marjoram (⅓ cup)

3 tablespoons thyme (⅓ cup)

3 tablespoons parsley flakes (⅓ cup)

3 tablespoons sage (⅓ cup)

3 tablespoons celery seed (⅓ cup)

1 tablespoon ground mace (2 tablespoons)

2 teaspoons white pepper (4 teaspoons)

2 teaspoons black pepper (4 teaspoons)

2 teaspoons paprika (4 teaspoons)

1 teaspoon cayenne pepper (2 teaspoons)

Liven up any dish without salt! This spice blend is perfect for salads, meats, soups, and casseroles. Grind it very fine and keep in a salt shaker on the table. You'll want more!
*Yield:* About 2 and 4 cups.

*Ultimate Poultry Seasoning*

⅓ cup basil (⅔ cup)

⅓ cup marjoram (⅔ cup)

⅓ cup thyme (⅔ cup)

¼ cup garlic powder (½ cup)

¼ cup onion powder (½ cup)

¼ cup smoked paprika (½ cup)

¼ cup salt (½ cup)

3 tablespoons savory (¼ cup)

3 tablespoons rosemary (¼ cup)

2 tablespoons black pepper (¼ cup)

No self-respecting bird would want to be cooked without this savory blend of herbs and spices! For a nice change of flavor, sprinkle some of this blend on veggies, fish, or even beef. *Yield:* About 2 ½ and 5 ¼ cups.

### *Crispy Refrigerator Dills*

½ cup kosher salt (1 cup)

½ cup dried minced garlic (1 cup)

½ cup whole dill seed (1 cup)

¼ cup whole coriander (½ cup)

¼ cup whole celery seed (½ cup)

¼ cup whole mustard seed (½ cup)

¼ cup ground cumin (½ cup)

3 tablespoons red pepper flakes (⅓ cup)

2 tablespoons ground turmeric (¼ cup)

2 tablespoons ground bay leaf (¼ cup)

This spicy, tangy recipe makes the best refrigerator pickles ever! To make, bring 5 cups water and 3 cups white vinegar to a boil and remove from heat. Stir in ¼ cup white sugar and 4–6 tablespoons seasoning mix. Cool completely. Pack freshly cut cucumbers into a jar and cover with brine. Refrigerate for one week before eating. One recipe yields 1 gallon of pickles. *Yield:* About 2 ¾ and 5 ½ cups.

Store bulk spice blends in glass jars with tight-fitting lids until you are ready to package them into decorative gifts. To do this you will need a funnel, lidded spice jars, labels, and some decorative packaging. Spice jars come in many sizes, and the following chart may help you decide which jar best suits your needs.

8 ounces = 16 tablespoons

6 ounces = 14 tablespoons

5 ounces = 11 tablespoons

4 ounces = 9 ½ tablespoons

2 ounces = 4 tablespoons

Repurposing the glass spice jars in which you purchased your individual spices saves time and money. Simply wash and remove the labels. Decorate the lids and hide any unwanted printing. Spray-paint the outer surfaces only. The inner portion of the lid should never be painted. As a finishing touch, decorate the jars with customized labels that include the name of the spice blend and the types of dishes it can be used for.

A small, decorative cardboard recipe box makes a nice presentation, as does a small spice rack. A fun and creative packaging option is a stainless steel tabletop salt and pepper holder. These usually come with empty shakers that you can fill with your homemade spice blends. By creating and sharing your own seasoning blends, you will be giving a wonderful, timeless, and much appreciated gift of spice.

# The Generous Geranium

≈ by Dallas Jennifer Cobb ≈

The Geranium is an annual flower commonly used in beds and pots to add visual color and texture to gardens. Because this annual is so commonly used for visual effect, its other uses are often overlooked. Did you know that Geraniums are edible?

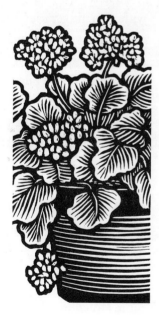

With so many different types of Geraniums available, their textures, scents, flavors, and colors make them a versatile ingredient in baking, salads, condiments, and drinks. Not only do Geraniums add their delicate scent and taste to culinary preparations, but their color makes for stunning food and drink presentation.

# About Geraniums

Geraniums are part of the *Geraniaceae* genus, and scented Geraniums are part of the *Pelargonium* species family. They are native to South Africa and the Cape of Good Hope. While scented Geraniums are perennial in those warm climates, in much of the United States and Canada they are considered annuals or tender perennials.

Varieties of Geraniums vary widely. Their leaves can be smooth, fuzzy like velvet, or even slightly tacky to the touch. The back of the leaf is the source of the Geranium's scent, where small glandular hairs secrete scented compounds, many of which are harvested for distillation into essential oils.

There are many different scented Geraniums available, with over fifty varieties of rose; many different lemon scents; varied fruit scents including apple, apricot, pineapple, and peach; and spice-scented Geraniums such as ginger, nutmeg, and cinnamon. While these scented varieties are often used in food and drink, please be aware that Citronella-scented Geranium is not edible and should not be used in consumables.

The Geranium's variety name usually denotes the flowers' scent and flavor, but don't be fooled by "Chocolate Mint Geranium." While it has a chocolaty brown color on its leaves, there is no chocolate taste, just fresh and cool mint. The lemon varieties of Geranium all have a crisp citrus smell and taste, and the other fruit flavors are delicate but distinct.

There are many varieties of Geraniums available through greenhouses and flower shops. When you first start to use Geraniums in your culinary creations, it's best to choose a few versatile varieties to grow and use. I recommend three versatile Geraniums for your use, which I will discuss later in this article.

A narrowed focus will save you money and garden space. With a basic knowledge of the appearance, color, and texture of a few common varieties, you can easily decide which ones will best suit your ongoing needs and tastes. Then, once you begin to develop your own recipes containing the generous Geranium, you may want to plant a Geranium garden devoted to the wide variety of available species. It will certainly be colorful, fragrant, and varied.

## General Geranium Info

Because Geraniums do well in dry heat and tolerate occasional watering, they are easy plants to grow. They love to be in pots, so are easy to keep on a balcony or porch, and usually do best in a pot that is almost too small for them. Geraniums don't like regular feeding, so skip the fertilizer and limit the compost. Give them slightly sandy soil, and even stick them in a planter with a bunch of other plants. Thriving on competition, dry soil, and pseudo-neglect, they will bloom faithfully until first frost.

This tender perennial will not survive a frost. Geraniums are also very hard to germinate from seed, so either take them inside and place them in a southern-facing window where they will bloom throughout most of the winter, or if you don't like the long legs that this produces, then take a cutting, root it in water, and plant it in soil to start a new plant indoors.

You can also cut Geraniums back drastically and put them in a very cool, dark basement for the winter months. When you bring them out in the spring, place them in direct sunlight, give them a little fresh compost to stimulate growth, and watch for the somewhat dormant roots to begin to sprout.

# Three Versatile Scented Geraniums

I keep three of the most versatile Geranium varieties on hand for cooking. The three I have chosen, and mention here, have three very different looking blooms, distinct leaves, and their own unique taste. These qualities make them a versatile flavor to add to food, and also provide a variety of colored blooms to add visual appeal to a meal.

My three favorite varieties are Rose Geranium (*Pelargonium graveolens*), which has gray-green leaves with triangular teeth on their edges, and pale pink flowers; the Lemon Fancy Scented Geranium (*Pelargonium crispum*), which has a strong lemon scent, deep dissected leaves, and pink blooms with a little spot of red in the middle; and the infamous Chocolate Mint Scented Geranium (*Pelargonium cv.*), which has gorgeous brown, chocolate-veined leaves that fan out in little hand shapes, and white flowers.

In the language of flowers from the Victorian era, each of these varieties has its own meaning. Rose represents desire, preference, and love; lemon represents tranquility of mind, unexpected delight, and good tidings; and peppermint is a wish for good health, energy, and vitality. Not only do these three varieties taste and look different, but they carry very different meanings or intention.

## Cooking with Geraniums

The general guideline for cooking with Geraniums is to "harvest" the flavor of the Geranium, but leave the leaves. Geranium leaves are tough and very fibrous, and while they are pretty, they are hard to eat. Because of this, the common use for the leaves is to immerse them in either oil, vinegar, or sugar and let them steep for a few weeks, absorbing the flavor and scent of the plant. The flavored oil or vinegar is then used for cooking, salad dressings, and meat seasoning, and the flavored sugar is commonly used in baking recipes.

You can also make tasty jellies or preserves out of the flavored leaves, so long as you strain out the fiber before canning. Many people have taken to making flavored Geranium tea from the leaves by pouring boiling water over them, allowing the mixture to steep, then straining out the leaf matter. This works well for either hot or cold infused beverages.

My grandmother used to make an Upside Down Apple and Rose Geranium Cake in which she layered Geranium leaves and sugar on the bottom of the pan, poured the batter over, and baked. When the cake was complete and cooled, she flipped it over onto a serving plate and carefully peeled off the leaves. Imagine the heavenly Rose scent and delicate imprint of leaves gracing the top of the cake—a gorgeous smell and a wonderful taste. I have included the recipe later in this article for your enjoyment.

## Scented Geranium Infusion Method

To steep in oil, vinegar, sugar, or water, place clean, dry scented Geranium leaves in a large sealable container. Sugar works well in a kitchen canister or Tupperware, while oil, vinegar, and water work best in a sealable glass container.

Layer the bottom of the sealable container loosely with leaves, then add your chosen medium so it covers the leaves entirely. Seal and label the jar with the ingredients and the date. Leave it at room temperature for two to four weeks. When you open the jar, carefully sieve the contents to remove the leaves, discarding them.

Scented oil and vinegar can be used to prepare tasty salad dressings and will keep in the refrigerator for a long time. Infused sugar will last almost indefinitely, and you can leave the leaves in the portion you are not using. The longer the leaves stay in, the stronger the scent and flavor of the Geraniums.

## Get Cooking

Whether you use infused ingredients, or simply use and then remove the leaves directly from your baking, you'll enjoy an enticing scented Geranium flavor in your recipes. With a bit of practice you can start to incorporate the scented Geranium infusions into all of your favorite recipes.

The Geranium is truly generous, lending its delicate scent and taste to all sorts of edible treats. Here are a few easy favorites to get you started. I urge you to go on and enjoy the generous Geranium.

## Scented Geranium Recipes

**Beverages**

*Scented Geranium Tea*

Take 12 scented Geranium leaves (use Lemon, Mint, or Rose, or try combining any two), crush lightly, and place in a 4-cup teapot. Pour boiling water over them and steep for 5 minutes. Serve with scented Geranium sugar, and enjoy. If you prefer iced tea, then steep the infusion and cool. Serve over ice with a Geranium leaf for garnish.

*Scented Geranium Lemonade*

⅓ cup scented Geranium sugar

6 cups water

½–¾ cup fresh squeezed lemon juice

8 scented Geranium leaves

Mix all ingredients carefully in a large jug. Pour over ice and serve. This summer favorite is made gourmet with the inclusion of Lemon or Mint scented Geranium sugar and leaves.

## Baked Treats

### *Lemon Geranium Scones*

Preheat oven to 425°F. Lightly oil a baking sheet.

3 cups flour

⅓ cup Lemon Geranium infused sugar

1 ½ teaspoons baking powder

½ teaspoon baking soda

¾ teaspoon salt

1 ½ sticks cold unsalted butter

1 cup milk

1 tablespoon grated lemon zest

Combine all the dry ingredients, then add the butter in small pieces and mix with your fingers. Add the milk and lemon zest, mixing well. Shape into 3-inch circles and bake for 10–12 minutes until golden brown. Serve hot with butter, Lemon Curd (recipe follows), or marmalade for a delightful treat.

### *Luscious Lemon Geranium Curd*

4 lemons

1 ½ cups Lemon Geranium infused sugar

1 stick unsalted butter at room temperature

4 extra-large eggs, also at room temperature

⅛ teaspoon salt

8 ramekin dishes

8 Lemon Geranium petals

Use a vegetable peeler or zester to "zest" the lemons (remove the peel in thin, slivery strips). Set zest aside, then cut the lemons in half and squeeze, gathering about ½ cup of juice. Set juice aside.

Put lemon zest and infused sugar in a food processor and mix for a minute or two until the zest is very fine. Add butter to the infused sugar and lemon zest, and cream. Add eggs, one at a time, while you continue mixing, then add lemon juice and salt. Mix well until ingredients are fully combined.

Pour the mixture into a medium saucepan and cook over low heat, stirring constantly, until it thickens in about 8–10 minutes. Remove from heat, and carefully fill the ramekin dishes with warm lemon curd. Decorate with a pretty Lemon Geranium petal on top. Allow the curd to set at room temperature.

### Lemon Geranium Pound Cake

½ cup butter, melted

1 cup Lemon Geranium infused sugar

2 eggs, well beaten

1 tablespoon lemon juice

¼ teaspoon salt

1 ½ cups flour

1 teaspoon baking powder

½ cup milk

⅓ cup lemon juice

¼ cup lemon zest (finely shaved lemon peel)

¼ cup Lemon Geranium infused sugar

Lemon scented Geranium petals, for garnish

Mix together 1 cup infused sugar and melted butter. Add eggs and 1 tablespoon lemon juice, and mix well. Add salt, flour, and baking powder. Add milk.

Bake mixture at 325°F in a well-greased loaf pan for 1 hour or until golden brown.

Mix ⅓ cup lemon juice, ¼ cup lemon zest, and ¼ cup Lemon Geranium infused sugar.

Use a toothpick to make holes in top of cake and drizzle lemon juice, lemon zest, and Lemon Geranium sugar mixture over the top of the cake when removed from the oven. Garnish with fresh Lemon scented Geranium petals, and serve warm or cool.

### Rose Geranium Scottish Shortbread Cookies

1 pound butter

½ cup Rose Geranium infused sugar

4 cups flour

1 cup cornstarch

24 Rose Geranium petals

Preheat oven to 300°F. Lightly oil a baking sheet.

Cream butter and infused sugar, then add cornstarch and flour gradually, kneading well with the palms of your hands. Press the mixture onto the baking sheet so it is about one-inch thick, then gently prick the surface with a fork. Bake slowly at 300°F for 45 minutes, then at 275°F for 1 hour, totaling 1¾ hours. Remove from oven, cut in squares, and let cool. Scatter with Rose Geranium petals and serve.

*Upside Down Apple and Rose Geranium Cake*

¼ cup butter

½ cup Rose Geranium infused sugar

1 egg, beaten

1 teaspoon vanilla

1 ½ cups flour

2 teaspoons baking powder

¼ teaspoon salt

½ cup milk

½ cup Rose Geranium infused sugar, for apples

4 apples, cored and sliced (many prefer to peel the apples, but I love the taste and texture of the peel)

1 cup Rose Geranium leaves

Rose Geranium petals, for garnish

Preheat oven to 325°F. Oil a large cake pan (9" x 12" or so).

Cream butter and ½ cup infused sugar, adding the vanilla and egg. In a separate bowl, combine the flour, baking powder and salt thoroughly, then add to the butter and sugar mixture, mixing well. Add milk. Cover the bottom of the baking dish with Rose Geranium leaves. Add a thin layer of infused sugar, then place half of the sliced apples on the bottom of the pan and cover with remaining sugar. Add another layer of apples, and cover everything with the cake batter. Bake for 40–45 minutes or until golden brown. When cool, flip cake over onto a serving platter, and carefully remove the Geranium leaves. Serve with a scatter of Rose Geranium petals.

# Delicious Dishes Featuring Fruits and Herbs

### ⤜ by Alice DeVille ⤛

When most consumers talk about favorite fruits, they mention the apple a day that keeps the doctor away, flavorful seasonal fruit salads, tart sauces such as traditional cranberry, or tempting dessert pies heaped with plump, juicy berries. Very few cooks think of reaching for herbs to enhance their fruit-based or fruit-accented dishes. Traditional fruit presentations fit easily on routine menus, yet adding only a few unexpected ingredients helps produce memorable new taste sensations.

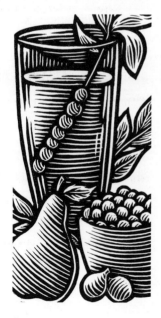

## Culinary License

Most chefs look for opportunities to modify, substitute, and create their own version of the standards. It's an intuitive thing. When cooks work with recipes, they often find ways to make them more distinctive. That's the approach I use after reading a recipe and deciding I want to add it to my repertoire. If it has possibilities but sounds bland, I find ways to make it more memorable by tweaking the ingredients. Experimentation leads to recipe invention. Foods go from good to great when you dare to be different in how you prepare your everyday meals. Salad fixings, suppers, and entrées come to life with new presentation options. Spreads and desserts burst with fresh fruit flavor artfully enhanced with garden herbs and lively spices.

This article challenges you to awaken the palates of friends and family by preparing main dishes, desserts, sauces, beverages, and appetizers with an infusion of interesting accent combinations. You'll find tips for giving favorite foods a flavor pick-me-up through integrating fruits and herbs into trusted recipes. Most don't take very long to prepare; some can be made ahead to save time on busy days. You're bound to find a new favorite.

## Wetting Your Whistle

**Spicy Blueberry Lemonade (makes 12 cups)**

- 2 pints blueberries, stemmed and rinsed, plus additional for garnish

- 2 cups sugar (or favorite substitute such as Stevia or Sweet'n Low)

- 2 quarts plus 2 cups water

- ½ cup basil leaves, packed, plus more for garnish

One 3-inch piece peeled ginger root, cut crosswise into thin slices (use half the amount of ginger if you find it too strong)

Finely grated zest and freshly squeezed juice of 4 to 5 lemons (4 tablespoons zest and 1 ½ cups juice)

Combine blueberries, sugar, and 2 cups of water in a large saucepan over medium heat. Cook for 4–5 minutes, stirring until the sugar dissolves and the berries just begin to burst. Cool slightly.

Transfer to the blender, along with the basil, ginger, and lemon zest. Purée until smooth, then strain into a pitcher or very large bowl, pushing the solids with a rubber spatula to extract all of the liquid. Discard solids.

Add the remaining 2 quarts of water and the lemon juice to the base mixture.

Serve over ice, mixing first with a half cup of club soda or seltzer per serving. Garnish the glass with blueberries threaded on a long skewer and basil or mint leaves, if desired.

*Note:* Many individuals find this core recipe without club soda too strong, while others use it as the base for alcoholic beverages. To make a cocktail, add gin or vodka and serve on the rocks or with a splash of club soda. Try making this lemonade with blackberries using a few variations: strain and discard the seeds along with the other solids; if you like a more intense color, add 1–2 drops blue food color to the liquid. Refrigerate until ready to serve, then mix with club soda and pour over ice. Use lemon-lime soda if you're up for a taste variation.

# Condiment with Class

Looking for an interesting new sandwich spread or a zesty fruit dip? Try this easy recipe on your favorite club sandwich, a BLT, or a chicken pita. Or serve it in a bowl with apple, peach, and pear slices, plus sharp cheese and crackers. If you prefer a dip, add ½ cup finely grated sharp cheese to the spread and serve with preferred accompaniments.

*Pear Mayonnaise (original recipe)*

    1 large ripe pear

    1 cup mayonnaise

    3 teaspoons Dijon mustard

    ¼ teaspoon each of minced parsley, basil, rosemary, and thyme, if using dried herbs; or increase to ½ teaspoon each if using fresh herbs, and mince finely

    For extra zip, add a few drops of hot sauce and blend before serving

Peel and core the pear and cut into quarters.

Put pear and all other ingredients in blender and pulse rapidly to combine. Spoon into small bowl if serving as a dip, or spread on slices of bread and add your favorite sandwich fillings, top with lettuce, and serve.

# Elegant Entrée

Main dishes go from ordinary to extraordinary with zesty touches that add no additional calories but enhance the taste. Here's a salmon dish that comes in at approximately 350 calories per serving.

### Panko-Ginger Salmon With Mango Peach Salsa
### (4 servings)

- 1 cup cubed peaches (½-inch pieces)
- 2 cups cubed mango (½-inch pieces)
- ¼ cup packed fresh cilantro leaves, finely chopped (may substitute with Italian parsley)
- 2 tablespoons fresh mint leaves, finely chopped
- 1 small jalapeño chile, stemmed, seeded, and finely chopped
- 2 tablespoons fresh lime juice
- Salt and pepper
- 2 teaspoons curry powder
- 2 tablespoons grated peeled fresh ginger
- ¾ cup Panko bread crumbs
- 4 pieces skinless salmon fillet (6 ounces each)
- 5 tablespoons vegetable oil

In medium bowl, combine peaches, mango, cilantro, mint, jalapeño, lime juice, and ¼ teaspoon salt, stirring until well mixed. Set aside.

In small bowl, stir together ginger, curry powder, Panko bread crumbs, ¼ teaspoon salt, and ½ teaspoon freshly ground black pepper. Add 3 teaspoons oil and mix well. Spread mixture evenly all over one side of each salmon fillet.

In nonstick grill pan, heat remaining oil on medium for 1 minute. Add salmon Panko side down and cook 10 minutes until salmon just turns opaque in center, turning over once. Cook other side another 3 minutes or until done. Top salmon with mango peach salsa.

*Note:* Make this dish when melons are in season by substituting the peaches with 1 cup honeydew and the mango with 2 cups cantaloupe.

## The Dinner Sandwich

The perception of sandwiches as a main dinner course conjures up a blah image when the family arrives home and asks *What's for dinner?* You won't get much of a cheer if you hand members a loaf of bread and suggest they build it themselves. Ingredients, condiments, and texture make a difference. With a little innovation on a day when you just don't have the energy to cook, debunk the myth and serve a hearty gourmet sandwich that says "wow" instead of "boring." Try this one on for size.

*Turkey-Havarti Sandwich with Spinach, Cherries, and Pears (serves 4)*

 1 small red onion cut into very thin slices

 1 tablespoon sugar

 Kosher salt to taste

 ¼ cup red wine vinegar

 ¼ teaspoon Herbes de Provence

 8 thick slices crusty multigrain or sourdough bread

 ¼ cup whole grain mustard

 4 ounces Havarti cheese (plain rather than dill- or peppercorn-infused—may substitute with smoked Gouda or Jarlsburg for a sharper bite)

 ¾ pound thinly sliced roasted turkey breast

 3 cups baby spinach leaves, stems removed

1 cup pitted dark-red cherries, coarsely chopped or
   mashed

8 slices d'Anjou or Bartlett pear

Mix the onion, sugar, a generous sprinkling of Kosher salt (approximately 1 teaspoon), and Herbes de Provence in a medium bowl; let sit for 5–10 minutes or until the onion wilts. Stir in the vinegar; let sit for another 10–15 minutes while the vinegar infuses the onions with flavor and the salt and sugar completely dissolve.

When you are ready to assemble the sandwiches, top 4 slices of the bread with a thin coating of Dijon or spicy whole grain mustard (you may also use the pear mayonnaise recipe listed earlier). In the following order, place the remaining ingredients in layers: turkey slices, cheese, some spinach leaves, a tablespoon of cherries (well drained), and 2 slices of pear. Top each portion with the remaining slices of bread spread with more mustard or a thin coating of pear mayonnaise. You may also omit any other condiment on the sandwich top. Cut in half. Serve immediately or assemble no more than an hour or two ahead of time to avoid the leaching of fruit liquid. I suggest experimenting with this recipe by excluding the cherries if you find that two fruits overpower the sandwich base. (This recipe was adapted from the collection of food expert Tony Rosenfeld.)

## Versatile Main Dish

Preparing meat dishes with fruit and wine pampers your taste buds and keeps your entrée moist and tender without raising the calorie count. Adding herbs and spices brings out the best flavors when the ingredients merge and appeal to your taste buds. The following flexible recipe works especially well with pork chops, turkey chops, and chicken or turkey cutlets. Fans of osso buco, veal chops, or veal cutlet will be pleased to know these meats work just as well—the secret is in the flavorful sauce. Whichever type of meat you prefer, be sure to tenderize it by pounding on each side with a meat mallet and then follow the remaining directions for preparing this succulent recipe. If you don't keep brandy on hand and don't want to purchase a bottle for use in this dish, you may substitute it with white grape juice or apple cider.

### Pork Chops with Green Grapes (4 servings)

4 six-ounce boneless pork chops about ¾-inch thick

1 tablespoon olive oil or more as needed

¼ cup flour

Kosher salt

Freshly ground black pepper to taste

1 sprig thyme, stem removed

2 large shallots

1 cup seedless green grapes cut in half if large

¼ cup dry white wine

2 teaspoons brandy (or substitute with white grape juice or apple cider)

1 cup low sodium chicken broth

1 ½ teaspoons dark brown sugar

1 tablespoon Dijon mustard

1 teaspoon butter (optional)

Trim off and discard any excess fat from the pork chops or other meat choice. After pounding the chops with a meat mallet, place them in a resealable plastic food storage bag along with the flour, salt, thyme leaves, and pepper. Seal the bag and shake to coat the meat evenly.

Meanwhile, heat the oil in a large cast-iron skillet over medium heat.

Shake off any excess flour from the pork chops and place them in the hot skillet. Cook for 4 minutes until lightly browned, then turn them over and cook for another 4 minutes. Transfer to a plate.

While the chops are cooking, mince the shallots to yield 4–5 tablespoons. Cut the grapes in half lengthwise. Combine the wine and brandy, if using, in a liquid measuring cup.

Reduce the heat to medium low. Add the shallots and grapes to the skillet. Cook for 4 minutes, stirring occasionally, then increase the heat to high and slowly add the wine mixture to the skillet being careful to avoid a flare-up from the alcohol. Cook for about 2 minutes or until the liquid evaporates.

Add the broth and brown sugar. Cook for about 2 minutes or until the liquid has been reduced by half.

Return the pork chops to the skillet. Cook for 2 minutes or until they are just heated through, turning them over as needed. Place the chops with some grapes on individual plates.

Whisk the mustard into the remaining liquid in the skillet to form an emulsified sauce.

*Optional:* At this point I often add 1 teaspoon butter because it makes the sauce taste succulent, and whisk again. Pour equal portions of the sauce over each pork chop. Serve warm.

Serve with a side dish of wilted spinach that has been combined with ¼ teaspoon crushed red pepper, ¼ teaspoon salt,

2–3 grinds of black pepper, and 2 teaspoons olive oil. Go for a full feast and add a side of mini farfalle or fusilli (½ cup per serving) that has been lightly tossed with butter or olive oil. Top with the chop and sauce and enjoy every savory morsel. Source: Main recipe adapted from *Melissa's Everyday Cooking with Organic Produce* by Cathy Thomas (Wiley, 2010).

# Dessert du Jour

Fibrous foods, especially those rich in color, have the most nutrition. Blackberries, with their deep purple shade, come loaded with more antioxidants than any other berry and are rich in vitamin C. You can prepare this tasty parfait in minutes while guests enjoy the conversation between courses.

*Purple Passion Parfait (4 servings)*

2 cups fresh, ripe blackberries, rinsed and drained

¼ cup sugar

1 cup crumbled shortbread, lemon cookies, or biscotti (store bought or home baked)

½ teaspoon very finely chopped fresh rosemary leaves (cut amount in half if using dried)

2 cups frozen vanilla yogurt (or vanilla ice cream, if you prefer)

Combine blackberries and sugar. Let stand 15 minutes.

With hands, mix cookie crumbles with fresh rosemary leaves.

Using 4 parfait glasses, layer berries, cookie crumbs, and frozen yogurt. Decorate with a mint sprig. Serve immediately.

# Pour It On:
# Herbal Sauces and Dips

### ❧ by Elizabeth Barrette ❧

Sauces, dips, and similar condiments provide a way of making simple foods more interesting. Although it's possible to load them with unhealthy ingredients, it's just as possible to make delicious condiments with herbs, fruits, vegetables, and other healthy things. Usually a condiment begins with a base, such as cream cheese, tomatoes, or oil, to which the flavorings are added.

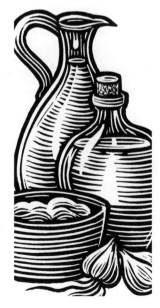

Always choose the best and freshest ingredients you can find for preparing sauces and dips. They will taste better and provide more nutrition. When you make your own condiments, you know exactly what goes into them and what doesn't. Commercial ones often include unappetizing ingredients such as high fructose corn syrup or MSG. They also tend to contain too much salt and sugar.

When making sauces and dips, you can use fresh or dried herbs. While it's possible to substitute one for the other, most recipes work better one way. You'll usually see recipes with all fresh herbs or all dried. Sometimes there will be dried herbs and spices mixed in, with a topping of fresh chopped herbs. Make sure the herbs you use are clean, and remove any yellowed or dirty leaves.

Cooking with herbs is easier if you have some special equipment. A mortar and pestle will be useful for hand-grinding things like peppercorns. For making pesto you need a larger mortar and pestle. A spice grinder or small coffee grinder is good for grinding small hard spices but can also be used to process fresh ginger root. If you want your sauces and dips to be perfectly smooth, you'll need a whisk, strainer, and/or blender. Immersion blenders can be stuck right into a pot to purée cooked vegetables and are thus very convenient.

# The Recipes

### Chocolate-Ginger Dip

    4 ounces dark chocolate

    1 inch fresh ginger root (about 1 tablespoon grated)

    ⅔ cup whole milk

    ⅓ cup heavy whipping cream

    ½ teaspoon powdered ginger

Grate the dark chocolate into a small bowl and set aside. Peel and grate 1 inch of fresh ginger root, which should yield about a tablespoon of grated ginger. Put in a small bowl and set aside.

Combine the whole milk and heavy whipping cream in a pot. Heat gently on the stove; do not allow to boil.

Slowly sprinkle the grated chocolate into the milk, stirring until the chocolate melts. Stir in the grated ginger. Finally, add ½ teaspoon powdered ginger.

Chocolate-ginger dip is excellent on fresh fruits, dried apricots or dried apples, cookies, sponge cake, or ice cream. You can even use it on pieces of candied ginger, candied angelica, or candied rose petals. If you want it to be completely smooth, you can use 1 teaspoon ginger juice instead of the grated ginger root. For extra zing, sprinkle candied ginger chips over the top of the dip.

### Cream Cheese Dip

1 package (8 ounces) cream cheese

1 cup milk

¼ teaspoon fine sea salt

¼ teaspoon white peppercorns

¼ teaspoon green peppercorns

3 garlic cloves

12 fresh chive leaves

Set the cream cheese on the counter to soften. Pour the cup of milk into a medium bowl, then stir in the fine sea salt. With a mortar and pestle, grind together the white and green peppercorns. Add the ground pepper to the milk and salt. Set aside.

Peel and mince the garlic cloves, then place them in a small bowl. Bundle the chive leaves together. Use kitchen scissors to snip the chives in tiny pieces over the bowl with the minced garlic. Set aside.

Put the softened cream cheese in a medium bowl. Gradually blend in the milk until the mixture is smooth and creamy. Then gently fold in the garlic and chives until fully combined.

This dip is good with corn chips, potato chips, or raw vegetables. To dress it up for a party, you can make a cream cheese log. Reduce milk to ½ cup. Oil a sheet of waxed paper and put the herbed cream cheese on it, then roll up the paper to shape the cream cheese into a log. Coat the log with chopped chives or chopped nuts, then refrigerate it to set before serving.

### Dried Herb Vinaigrette

> ¾ cup extra-virgin olive oil
>
> ¼ cup red wine vinegar
>
> ¼ teaspoon pink salt (Himalayan, Australian, etc.)
>
> ¼ teaspoon rose baises peppercorns
>
> ¼ teaspoon black peppercorns
>
> 1 garlic clove
>
> ½ teaspoon dried thyme
>
> ½ teaspoon rubbed sage
>
> ¼ teaspoon ground rosemary

In a small mixing bowl, whisk together the olive oil and red wine vinegar.

With a mortar and pestle, grind together the pink salt, rose baises peppercorns, and black peppercorns. Add to the mixing bowl and whisk ingredients again.

Peel and mince the garlic clove and add it to the mixing bowl. Add the dried thyme, rubbed sage, and ground rosemary. Whisk thoroughly.

Pour the vinaigrette into a bottle and store in the refrigerator at least overnight to allow the flavors to blend. Shake before serving. Pour over a mixed salad such as baby lettuces, baby spinach, French sorrel, and so on. This can also be used as a marinade for meats before they are cooked.

## Pesto Sauce

1 large bunch of fresh basil leaves (3–4 cups)

4 garlic cloves

2 ounces Parmesan cheese

¼ teaspoon sea salt

½ teaspoon green peppercorns

¼ cup pine nuts (pignolia)

½ cup extra-virgin olive oil

Rinse and dry the basil. Tear the leaves into small pieces, discarding any tough stems or damaged parts, and put the torn leaves in a medium bowl. Peel and mince the garlic cloves. Add the minced garlic to the torn basil. Set aside.

Grate the Parmesan cheese into a small bowl and set aside.

Grind the sea salt and green peppercorns together with a mortar and pestle. Add the pine nuts and grind again.

Put the basil and garlic into the mortar and pestle and grind to paste. (This will take a while.) Add the grated Parmesan cheese and grind that in. Slowly add the olive oil and whisk the pesto so it blends evenly.

Pesto sauce is excellent on pasta or pizza and also goes well with fish or chicken. If you don't have a mortar and pestle, you can make the pesto in a blender or food processor, but it will turn out runnier and the flavor isn't quite as good. For an interesting twist, you can use a purple variety of basil.

*Spaghetti Sauce with Mushrooms and Herbs*

    4 celery ribs

    1 red onion

    1 bell pepper

    ¼ cup olive oil

    3 pounds red beefsteak tomatoes

    2 pounds ripe green tomatoes (Cherokee Green, German Green, Green Pineapple)

    8-ounce package of sliced mushrooms (golden or button)

    6 long sprigs of sweet marjoram (about 2 tablespoons)

    6 large leaves of sage (about 1 tablespoon)

    3 long sprigs of oregano (about 1 tablespoon)

    8–10 sprigs of thyme (about 2 teaspoons)

    1 handful of basil leaves (about ⅓ cup)

    4 garlic cloves (about 2 teaspoons minced)

    1 bay leaf

    1 teaspoon pink salt (Himalayan, Australian, etc.)

    ½ teaspoon rainbow assortment of peppercorns (black, white, pink, and green)

    24 ounces unseasoned tomato paste

2 tablespoons brown sugar

¼ cup molasses

Fill two large pots with water. Set one of them to boil for scalding the tomatoes.

Wash the celery ribs, cut off the ends, then slice into thin crescents. (If the bottom parts are really wide, cut stalk into thirds and split the lower thirds vertically before slicing.) Peel and chop the onion. Remove seeds and ribs from the bell pepper and chop it. Combine all vegetables in a medium bowl.

Pour the olive oil into a large crockpot. Add the mixed vegetables. Turn crockpot on low and cover.

Wash all the tomatoes. Remove the stems and score the sides. When water reaches a rolling boil, add tomatoes 2–3 at a time. Wait 30–60 seconds until skins begin to wrinkle and peel. Transfer tomatoes to cold water. Remove and discard skins. Chop the peeled tomatoes. Add them to the crockpot and stir.

Gather the sweet marjoram, sage, oregano, thyme, and basil leaves. Fold the marjoram sprigs into a loose cylinder; use kitchen scissors to snip the leaves into the crockpot. Next use the kitchen scissors to cut the sage leaves in half, removing large ribs. Stack the slices and snip into small bits over the crock pot. Strip the oregano leaves off the stems; discard stems. Wad the oregano leaves into a cylinder and snip them into the crockpot. Strip the thyme leaves off the stems and drop the leaves into the crockpot. Tear the basil leaves in half or quarters, removing large ribs. Roll them into a cylinder and snip into the crockpot. Then stir.

Peel and mince the garlic cloves and add to crockpot. Add the bay leaf and pink salt. With a mortar and pestle, grind the rainbow assortment of peppercorns. Add the ground pepper to crockpot and stir again.

Cook on low for about 4 hours. Stir, then taste. Add the unseasoned tomato paste. Stir carefully until fully blended. Cook another hour or so. Stir, then taste. The spaghetti sauce will probably be sour at this stage. Stir in the brown sugar and molasses. Cook for another hour or so.

At this point the sauce is built, though only partially cooked. To fine-tune the flavor, taste and pay careful attention to what is changing as the sauce cooks. If it tastes flat, try adding a little more salt and ground pepper. If it's still sour, add a bit more brown sugar. If the leafy notes from the herbs are not strong enough, add more, starting with the sage and oregano. Add one or two things at a time if needed, then wait half an hour for them to blend in properly. Continue stirring and tasting occasionally.

The sauce is done when (1) all the vegetables are translucent and tender; (2) the body of the sauce is thick, opaque, and deep red; and (3) you feel satisfied with the flavor. This takes about 8–10 hours total, depending on the crockpot.

Stir the sauce. Find and remove the bay leaf. If you are serving the sauce fresh, it can be poured over pasta or placed on the table for people to use as they wish. If you are storing it, pour the sauce into containers to refrigerate or freeze. This recipe makes about 9–10 cups of sauce. A 2 ½-cup carton of sauce poured over spaghetti will feed 3–4 people, so figure this recipe at 11–14 servings.

### Spicy Barbecue Sauce

    8 pounds sauce tomatoes (Roma, etc.)

    2 yellow onions

3 sweet bell peppers

2 hot peppers (habañero, Scotch bonnet, etc.)

8 garlic cloves

2 tablespoons olive oil

1 tablespoon smoked salt

1 teaspoon black peppercorns

8 dried juniper berries

1 teaspoon chipotle powder

½ teaspoon cinnamon

10 fresh garlic chive leaves

6 fresh sage leaves

4 fresh oregano sprigs

1 fresh rosemary sprig

1½ cups apple cider vinegar

1 cup brown sugar

Fill two large pots with water. Set one of them to boil for scalding the tomatoes.

Wash the tomatoes. Remove the stems and score the sides. When water reaches a rolling boil, add tomatoes 2–3 at a time. Wait 30–60 seconds until skins begin to wrinkle and peel. Transfer tomatoes to cold water. Remove and discard skins. Cut the tomatoes in half and carefully squeeze out as much of the seeds and juice as possible. Put the tomato halves in a colander to drain.

Peel and chop the onions. Rinse the bell peppers, then remove the stems, cores, and seeds. Chop the bell peppers. Rinse, core, and chop the hot peppers the same way. Peel and mince the garlic cloves. Put these vegetables in a medium bowl and set aside.

Put the olive oil into the bottom of a large pot, add the tomato halves, and set the stove to simmer. Add the bowl of chopped vegetables and stir.

With a mortar and pestle, combine the smoked salt, black peppercorns, and dried juniper berries. Grind together and add to the simmering tomatoes. Stir in the chipotle powder and cinnamon.

Gather the fresh garlic chive leaves, fresh sage leaves, fresh oregano sprigs, and fresh rosemary sprig. Using kitchen scissors, snip the chive leaves into the pot. Cut the sage leaves in half, remove the tough center ribs, and snip the leaves into the pot. Strip the leaves off the oregano sprigs; discard stems. Roll the leaves into a cylinder and snip over the pot. Strip the needles off the rosemary sprig; discard the stem. Pinch the needles together and snip over the pot. Stir everything together.

Add the apple cider vinegar and brown sugar. Stir again. Simmer gently for about half an hour, until vegetables soften and tomatoes begin to break down. Adjust seasonings for taste if necessary.

Run the cooked mixture through a food mill or canning sieve, or purée it with a blender. Next, pour the sauce into a crockpot and cook on low for 3–4 hours, stirring once every 30 minutes or so. Leave the lid ajar so steam can escape.

Allow the sauce to cook down until it reaches the consistency that you like your barbecue sauce to be. (Bear in mind that it will thicken a little more as it cools.) You can then use it fresh, can it, or freeze it for later use. This recipe makes about 4 pints of barbecue sauce, which is good on beef, pork, lamb, or game meats such as venison.

# The Perfect "Cuppa" Hot Chocolate

### ≈ by Susan Pesznecker ≈

While hot chocolate drinks are year-round favorites, they turn up most often during autumn and winter, especially when topped with whipped cream or a couple of giant marshmallows. We tend to use the terms hot cocoa and hot chocolate interchangeably, but they are actually two very different things. Hot cocoa is made from cocoa powder, which is a dry, powdered chocolate with the cocoa butter removed. In contrast, hot chocolate is made from solid chocolate that is melted into milk or cream. A world of variations spins off from these two basic forms, but one constant is that in every case, the higher quality the chocolate, the better the drink.

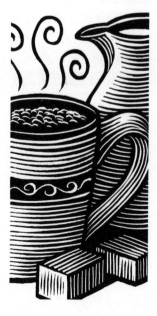

Hot chocolate comes with its own trove of lore and legend. The first hot chocolate beverage was credited to the Mayans, who drank bitter, unsweetened hot chocolate enhanced with spicy peppers. The drink was prized as a food of the gods and was used mostly by those of status; it was not necessarily a drink for commoners. The Aztecs, too, drank hot chocolate, and with the colonization of North America, the drink moved from Mexico into the rest of the continent and then spread to Europe. The rest is history.

Besides being a sacred drink often used in ritual or ceremony, hot chocolate has long had medicinal uses, particularly in treating gastrointestinal disorders. Scientists today have identified chocolate as a potent source of antioxidants which, when used moderately, may actually reduce the risk of heart disease. Chocolate also affects neurotransmitters in the brain and has been linked to improved mood and diminished depression. In J. K. Rowling's Harry Potter books, the characters ate chocolate to "keep the dementors away"—which sounds as if Rowling knew what she was talking about!

## The Chocolate

The chocolate, of course, is the most important ingredient in hot chocolate beverages. Splurge on the very best chocolate or cocoa powder you can afford, and for best results when following recipes, weigh the chocolate with a good food scale.

Cocoa powder—used in hot cocoa—comes in two basic varieties: regular and "Dutch" processed. Both are a powdered chocolate from which the cocoa butter has been removed. Dutch processed cocoa is further treated with an alkali to neutralize the chocolate's acidity; the result is somewhat smoother than plain cocoa powder. However, the Dutch process itself destroys many of the valuable antioxidants in the cocoa, reducing its healthful properties.

Chocolate—used in hot chocolate—may be labeled as milk, semisweet, unsweetened (also called "baking" chocolate), or dark (graded according to percent of cocoa solids). Milk chocolate is mild and sweet, and semisweet chocolate contains some sugar and has a stronger, mildly bitter flavor. Dark chocolate contains even less sugar than semisweet and at least 35 percent cocoa solids; the higher the percentage of cocoa solids, the darker and more intense the chocolate flavor. Unsweetened chocolate contains no sugar and doesn't taste very good on its own. Try it, though, so you'll know. For that matter, taste and experiment with all the different chocolates until you find those you like best.

Solid chocolate is available in chips, bars, and as ground chocolate. Although it looks much like cocoa, ground chocolate contains cocoa butter; you can use ground chocolate in your hot chocolate recipes interchangeably for solid chocolate. Chocolate syrup is something altogether different: a mixture of sugar, flavorings, stabilizers, and chemicals—not what we're discussing here.

## Milk, Sugar, and the Rest

Next to chocolate, the most important ingredient in hot chocolate drinks is milk. Any combination of milk and cream can be used to make hot chocolate or cocoa, and as a rule, the higher the fat content, the richer and creamier the result. Soy, rice, coconut, and other nondairy milks will work, too, with experimentation to adjust for their unique flavors.

Some recipes use cans of evaporated or sweetened condensed milk, and it's essential to know the difference. Evaporated milk is unsweetened milk with much of the water removed, leaving it slightly thickened. It can be used for hot chocolate or cocoa, usually diluted 2:1 or 1:1 with water. Sweetened condensed milk, on the other hand, is an ultra-condensed milk product with lots of sugar added, creating a dense, creamy, sticky product. If using sweetened condensed milk in hot chocolate and cocoa, avoid adding sugar until you've tasted the mixture.

Speaking of sugar, if you're using it in your hot chocolate drinks, add slowly and taste as you go. Virtually any sweetener will work, and some lend unique flavors. Consider white, brown, or raw sugar, as well as honey, agave syrup, or even maple syrup. If you're using artificial sweetener, add it just before serving to ensure the heat of the cooking process doesn't make it turn bitter.

Some basic equipment will help you brew the perfect cuppa chocolate. A one- or two-quart saucepan is the right size for small recipes. Measuring cups and spoons will help you measure ingredients, and a kitchen scale is invaluable for weighing chocolate—especially the expensive stuff. A small whisk is essential, both for stirring and frothing.

## Making Hot Cocoa

Hot cocoa is a mixture of milk, dry cocoa powder, and sugar. It's a delicious, homey drink, and one of its main advantages is that the ingredients are those one tends to have on hand in the kitchen. Cocoa powder has a long shelf life and is relatively inexpensive: a cup of homemade hot cocoa costs just pennies.

Best of all, hot cocoa is easy to make. When first added to the milk, the dry powdered cocoa will float on the surface and look like it's not going to cooperate with the process. But have no fear: the heat will quickly melt the cocoa and create a mug of steaming chocolatey goodness.

*Key Recipe: Hot Cocoa for One*

In a small saucepan, combine ¼ cup water, 2 teaspoons sugar, and 1 tablespoon cocoa powder. I like to use a dark chocolate cocoa powder. Whisk and stir over medium heat until the mixture is hot and the cocoa powder has melted, then whisk again until smooth.

Add 1 cup milk and a few drops of pure vanilla extract, and heat until steaming hot. I often add a pinch of cayenne, creating drinkable warmth all the way down to my toes. Whisk before serving to create a frothy surface.

## Making Hot Chocolate

Hot chocolate is pricier than cocoa—because of the fresh chocolate used—but it's well worth the expense. Making hot chocolate is simple. Heat milk over medium heat, stirring frequently so it doesn't stick or scorch. Melt the chocolate slowly in the steaming hot milk, whisking frequently as it melts. You can do this in the microwave, too, heating milk and chocolate in a large glass bowl or measuring cup and working in 20–30 second increments, stirring between each.

*Key Recipe: Hot Chocolate for One*

Follow the above instructions, using 1 cup milk and 1 ounce chocolate. I like to use 60 percent dark chocolate, adding 1 teaspoon sugar to the mixture; if you use milk or semisweet chocolate, you probably won't need or want the sugar. Just before serving, add a few drops of pure vanilla extract. My favorite topper is a dollop of whipped cream.

The beverage known as "drinking chocolate" is hot chocolate taken to new heights. Drinking chocolate has a much higher percentage of chocolate to milk and typically has less sugar, too. The resulting drink—served in very small portions—is somewhere between heavy cream and light pudding in texture. It is exquisite.

### Drinking Chocolate for Two ... or More

Follow the key recipe for "Hot Chocolate for One," but use 1 cup whole milk, ¼ cup heavy cream, 3 ounces high-quality solid chocolate, and 1 ½ tablespoons sugar. Just before serving, stir in ⅛ teaspoon vanilla extract. If desired, add ⅛ teaspoon cinnamon and a pinch of cayenne pepper. Divide among two or more small cups and top with whipped heavy cream. Enjoy!

## Toppers and Add-Ins

Spices and extracts can enhance your recipes. I add a bit of pure vanilla extract to all of my hot chocolate drinks: it tastes great and seems to balance out the chocolate's innate bitterness. Drops of rum, orange, and peppermint extracts create nice effects, too. A sprinkle of cinnamon is festive and lends a traditional Mexican feel to hot cocoa, while a tiny pinch of cayenne doesn't change the flavor but imparts a warmth that you'll feel deep down inside as you sip the hot drink. As for salt, I don't generally salt an individual mug of cocoa, but if stirring up a kettle for a crowd, I'll add a pinch of salt for balance.

The ultimate topping for hot chocolate is whipped heavy cream. And no, I don't mean those buckets of dessert topping found in the freezer case. Those are made of emulsified oils—not something you want melting into your cocoa! Buy good heavy cream—organic if you can find it. Whip ½ cup cold cream with a mixer in a chilled bowl until soft peaks form. Beat in ¼ teaspoon vanilla and 1 tablespoon confectioner's sugar until peaks stiffen more. Plop this atop your cocoa and prepare to be in heaven. Sprinkle the whipped cream with grated chocolate, cinnamon, crushed peppermint candy, nutmeg, or whatever else tickles your fancy. You can also stir in a spoon or two of liqueur or brandy while beating the cream.

Marshmallows are another classic hot cocoa topper, and recently marshmallow companies began coming out with bags of mallows in seasonal shapes and colors. Marshmallows add a lot of sweetness; if you know you're going to add them to your cocoa, you'll want to use less sugar in your recipe.

Add-ins can be wonderful additions to your hot chocolate, too. Replace some of the milk with strong hot coffee for a mocha flavor. Stir in orange peel, raspberry syrup, caramel syrup, or various liquors and liqueurs. Peppermint schnapps, coffee liqueur, and brandy are delightful embellishments. And, of course, you can buy commercial coffee syrups in a rainbow of flavors.

Add a cinnamon stick or candy cane stirrer to the mug of hot cocoa for a treat. For something really fun, dip a teaspoon in melted chocolate, then cool on waxed paper. Serve the cup of hot chocolate with the chocolate spoon on the side; dipped into the hot beverage, the chocolate melts and enriches the drink.

## Unusual Effects

White chocolate isn't actually chocolate but is a mixture of sugar, cocoa butter, and milk. It can make a sweet, wintery drink.

*Key Recipe: Hot White Chocolate for One*

In a small saucepan, combine 1 cup milk and 1–2 ounces white chocolate. Heat gently over medium heat, whisking frequently. Add a few drops of pure vanilla extract just before serving and top with mini marshmallows.

Two of my friends swear by adding butter to their hot cocoa. They smoosh a small amount of unsalted butter into the cocoa powder and sugar mixture, then proceed as usual. They tell me it adds a wonderful richness to the drink.

Making hot cocoa or chocolate for a crowd? Use your slow cooker to keep the drink steamy-perfect for hours. Imagine the fun of hosting a hot chocolate "bar," with a slow cooker full of cocoa and an array of toppers, stir sticks, and add-ins.

## Pre-Made Hot Chocolate

I've been mostly disappointed with the taste of commercial hot cocoa mixes. Here's an option for making your own mix.

*Key Recipe: Hot Cocoa Mix*

In a medium bowl, combine 2 ¾ cups powdered milk, 2 ounces powdered nondairy creamer, ½ cup confectioner's sugar, and 6 tablespoons cocoa powder. Blend well and store in a lidded jar. To use, stir 3–4 tablespoons mix into a cup of steaming hot water. Add additional sugar as desired.

*Variation:* Omit the powdered milk; use 1–2 tablespoons mix per cup of steaming water.

However you make it, enjoy your favorite cuppa chocolate. Stir it up in your kitchen, pour it into a favorite cup or mug, and enjoy the "drink of the gods." Now, if you'll excuse me, I hear a mug of hot, dark, peppered chocolate calling my name…

# Give Your Regards to Bay Leaves: The Kitchen's Most Underappreciated Herb

### ➤ by Anne Sala ➤

**B**oth noble and unassuming, necessary yet with elusive qualities, the bay leaf is a spice rack staple that is easy to take for granted. Once valued in many cultures for its medicinal, magical, and purifying properties, the bay leaf is now relegated to the kitchen. Even so, it continues to impart its considerable powers through every recipe that calls for it.

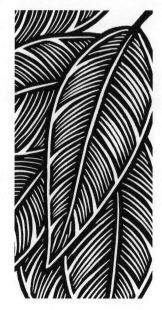

*Laurus nobilis*, known as bay, sweet bay, and laurel, is an evergreen tree that produces leathery, oval leaves. Tiny yellow flowers turn into dry, black, berry-like seeds when they mature. The tree is a popular container plant, but can also grow 25 feet tall in a favorable climate.

There are many varieties of bay throughout the world, but the ones originating in the Mediterranean are some of the most highly regarded for cooking. Along with sweet bay, golden and willow leaf bay are popular types used in the kitchen. To be assured that the bay you have is a member of the *Laurus nobilis* family, hold a leaf up to a light source. If the leaf is translucent, revealing its network of veins, and it gives off a rich scent when crushed, it is a true bay.

Greek mythology states the laurel tree was created when the nymph Daphne rejected the amorous advances of the god Apollo. As she ran from him, she cried for help and her father transformed her into the laurel tree. Despite this apparent rebuff, Apollo still loved her. He declared the bay to be one of his sacred emblems and took to wearing a wreath of laurel on his head.

Following Apollo's lead, Greeks and Romans crowned celebrated individuals with laurel wreaths. Recipients included the victors in battles and competitions, poets, and philosophers. This practice of crowning people with laurel is where the terms Poet Laureate and Nobel Laureate come from, as well as "resting on one's laurels" (meaning being satisfied with past success and no longer trying to improve oneself).

Emperors also wore laurel wreaths. Perhaps they did this to appear godlike, but it may also have been because the leaves were supposed to protect against lightning strikes.

Medically, bay is an important herb due to its astringent qualities. It can also be used as a diuretic and as an appetite stimulant. When rubbed into the skin, its essential oil helps treat bruises, sprains, and rheumatism.

Perhaps the bay leaf's ability to quell flatulence and aid in the digestion of greasy foods helped it migrate from a religious and medical tool to a culinary herb. Plus, the leaves dry well and have a long shelf life. In addition, the dried berries were once crushed and used to season food in a similar manner to black pepper.

Whether fresh or dried, bay leaves are tough and inedible when whole, but safe to consume when ground into powder. Ingesting large quantities of the herb, however, is not advised. It is said the Oracle of Delphi chewed bay leaves to induce her visions of the future.

The appearance of bay leaves in a recipe is rarely called into question, yet what flavor does this herb actually bring to the dish? At the same time, if the bay leaf was omitted, would it be missed? I say it would, but it might be tricky to pinpoint what exactly was missing.

Described as piney, sweetly spicy, and "aromatic," the taste of bay is hard to identify. It might be easier to portray its taste as a purpose. It fills out the flavor of the other ingredients in a dish and can transform a new recipe into your family's next comfort food. One could also say the bay leaf embodies the ambiguous term *umami*—a hard-to-describe yet satisfying "savory mouthfeel" that certain foods have.

In their article "The Noble Bay," authors Madalene Hill and Gwen Barclay call bay a "liaison" herb: "Like parsley and sweet marjoram, bay laurel helps other contrasting flavors blend together. We like to think that when one of these liaison herbs is used with other more assertive ones, the flavors don't fight one another."

# Bay Leaf Recipes

## Bouquet Garni

One of the most familiar uses of bay leaves is in a *bouquet garni*. Meaning "garnished bunch," it is a selection of herbs that are tied together, or enclosed in a porous container (like a cloth bag or tea strainer), and used to flavor a soup or casserole. The bundle is removed before serving.

Numerous combinations of herbs can be used in a bouquet garni, depending on the type of food it is seasoning, but the bay leaf is almost always included. Common mixtures include thyme, parsley, and bay for generally anything; rosemary, summer savory, hyssop, and bay for chicken; leek greens, parsley, tarragon, and bay for fish; and oregano, thyme, bay, and lovage (or celery) for red meat.

## Beef Stew with Dumplings

Putting the "liaison herb" theory to the test, bay leaves help the strong flavor of beef contend with the other robust herbs in this recipe. The dumplings, however, do better with a lighter touch, hence my instructions to season them with only one of the herbs present in the stew. This way, their buoyant nature is not dragged down by competing flavors. Serves 4 to 6.

*For the stew:*

    2 pounds beef rump roast, cut into ½-inch cubes

    1 pound red potatoes, cut into ½-inch cubes

    ½ pound yellow onions, chopped

    ½ pound carrots, cut into ½-inch pieces

    ½ cup red wine

    3–4 branches of oregano

    3–4 branches of thyme

3 large bay leaves

3–4 branches of lovage or one 4-inch stalk of celery

2 tablespoons or more all-purpose flour or more to coat

6 cups water

2–3 tablespoons vegetable oil

Salt and pepper to taste

*For the dumplings:*

2 cups all-purpose flour

3 teaspoons baking powder

1 teaspoon salt

2 teaspoons dried thyme or 3 teaspoons fresh thyme leaves

4 tablespoons butter, chilled

1 cup buttermilk, or mix 1 tablespoon vinegar into 1 cup milk and allow to stand for at least 5 minutes

1. Place a large pot or Dutch oven over medium heat. Film the bottom with vegetable oil.

2. Measure flour for beef stew into a small paper bag or gallon-size resealable plastic bag. Add meat and shake to coat.

3. Working in batches, brown the meat on all sides. Add oil and adjust the heat if necessary to prevent burning. Transfer cooked meat to a plate.

4. Meanwhile, make a bouquet garni. Use a tea ball or bundle up the bay leaves, oregano, thyme, and lovage or celery, and tie together with kitchen string. You can snip the extra string or leave a tail that you can tie to the pot handle to aid in its removal after you are done cooking. Set aside.

5. After the last of the meat has browned and is removed, deglaze the pot with the wine. Allow the wine to cook down for a couple minutes, then return the meat and any pooled juices to the pot.

6. Add the water and bouquet garni. Cover and simmer for 45 minutes.

7. Add the carrots, onions and potatoes. Season with salt and pepper. Cover and simmer for an additional 45 minutes, at which time the meat should be starting to break down. Also, the liquid level should have reduced enough to reveal bits of meat and vegetables above the surface, creating places for you to put the dumplings. If the liquid level is too high, increase the heat slightly and continue cooking without the lid to help the liquid reduce while you prepare the dumplings.

8. Mix together the dry dumpling ingredients and herbs in a large bowl.

9. Cut in butter, using two knives or your hands, until the dough is crumbly.

10. Stir in buttermilk, being careful not to overmix. Let stand for 5–10 minutes.

11. Using two teaspoons, drop the batter onto the stew, aiming for the exposed meat and vegetables.

12. Bring the stew back to a soft simmer and cook for 10 minutes with the lid off and then 10 minutes with the lid on.

13. Serve hot with red wine vinegar to sprinkle on the dumplings.

*Chicken and Rice Casserole with Apples and Bay*

This recipe is great on a crisp fall evening. It is a fine example of how bay leaves play well with both fruit and meat. While the cheese is optional, I recommend it. If the apples are organic, consider leaving the peels intact to add some color. Serves 4.

8 skinless, boneless chicken thighs

2–3 tart apples, peeled, cored, and sliced thin

1 medium onion, chopped

2 cups chicken or vegetable broth

1 cup uncooked rice

2 tablespoons butter

2 tablespoons all-purpose flour

¼ cup milk

1 tablespoon olive oil

3–4 dried bay leaves

Salt and pepper to taste

½ cup cheddar cheese, cubed (optional)

1. Place a lidded, ovenproof pan over medium heat. When the pan is hot, add oil and sauté onions. Preheat the oven to 375°F.

2. Melt butter in the pan, then stir in flour to create a roux.

3. Add milk and broth. Bring to a boil while stirring continuously until the sauce is smooth.

4. Remove the pan from heat. Place the apple slices in a single layer and sprinkle evenly with rice. Nestle the chicken thighs and bay leaves in the mixture. Season with salt and pepper.

5. Place lid on pan and bake for about 50 minutes, or until the thighs are cooked through and the liquid is absorbed.

6. Remove pan from oven and place on a heatproof surface. Dot the rice and chicken with the cheese. Replace the lid and let the cheese melt. Serve hot.

### Porgies and Bay

This dish is deceptively easy and is impressive to serve at a party. You can even prepare the seasoning ahead of time and store in the refrigerator. Serves 4 to 6.

Two one-pound porgies (or any other mild, white-fleshed fish), gutted and scaled

One 1-inch piece fresh ginger, finely minced

2 garlic cloves, minced

3 tablespoons red onion, minced

½ small jalapeño pepper, seeded and minced

¼ teaspoon ground star anise

1 tablespoon soy sauce

10 fresh bay leaves, split six of them in half lengthwise

1–2 tablespoons canola oil

Salt and pepper

1. Preheat oven to 375°F. Mix together ginger, garlic, onion, jalapeño, star anise, and soy sauce. Season with salt and pepper.

3. Rinse fish and dry with paper towels. Place them on an oiled baking sheet. Using a sharp knife, carefully make three slashes crosswise on both sides of each fish.

4. Use your fingers to stuff the seasoning mixture into the slashes and body cavities. Rub any that is left over on the skin.

Insert a bay leaf half into each of the slashes and place two whole bay leaves into each of the body cavities. Drizzle with oil.

5. Roast for at least 20 minutes, or until the flesh flakes. Serve immediately, drizzling each portion with some of the pan juices.

### Banana Bay Rice Pudding

Custards flavored with bay are a traditional dessert in England. Here, the alluring flavor is transferred to rice pudding. Also, the addition of the banana cuts down on the amount of sugar needed. Serves 4.

2 ½ cups milk, preferably whole

½ cup medium grain rice, such as arborio

½ cup sugar

⅛ teaspoon salt

1 very ripe banana, peeled and diced

2 dried bay leaves

1. Place all ingredients in a medium saucepan over high heat. Stir until sugar dissolves and the mixture comes to a boil.

2. Lower heat to keep the pudding at a simmer. Stir frequently until it is thick and the rice is tender, about 30–45 minutes, depending on the rice and type of milk used. Serve hot, warm, or cold.

### Bread Scented with Bay Leaves

I was inspired to make this bread after reading about how the Romans used to bake a special wedding pastry on a bed of bay leaves. Makes 2 loaves.

1 short tablespoon or 1 package active dry yeast

2 cups lukewarm water

1 tablespoon salt

½ teaspoon sugar

1–2 tablespoons olive oil

4–6 cups flour (you may use either all-purpose or bread flour)

6–8 bay leaves, either fresh or dried

Cornmeal

1. Mix yeast and warm water in a small bowl and stir in sugar. Let stand for at least 5 minutes. As the yeast activates, it should start to bubble up.

2. Pour the yeast mixture into a large bowl. Add salt and 2 cups of flour. Stir with a wooden spoon for about 2 minutes.

3. Continue stirring while incrementally adding flour. When the dough becomes too stiff to stir, begin kneading with your hands. The dough should be kneaded for at least 5 minutes until smooth in appearance and no longer sticky.

4. Place the dough in a medium-size bowl that has been coated with 1 tablespoon of the oil. Cover and let rise in a warm spot until it doubles in size, about 45 minutes.

5. Punch down the dough, divide in half, and let rest for 10 minutes. At this time you may place one piece (or both) of dough in a resealable plastic bag and store in the refrigerator to bake on a different day. Just allow the dough to return to room temperature before continuing with the recipe.

6. Grease a cookie sheet with the remaining oil and sprinkle with cornmeal. Decide if you are going to make a round bread loaf or a baguette, and arrange the bay leaves on the sheet so, in the next step, the dough will completely cover them.

7. Shape the dough and place on the cookie sheet, on top of the bay leaves. Cut 3–4 gashes in the top of the loaf and cover with a cotton tea towel. Allow the bread to rise until double in size.

8. Bake the bread in a 400°F oven for 30–40 minutes. The bread should sound hollow when tapped on the bottom. Remove bay leaves and cool the bread on a wire rack for at least 30 minutes before slicing.

## References

Beard, James. *Beard on Bread.* New York: Alfred A. Knopf, 1973.

Better Homes and Gardens. *Complete Guide to Food and Cooking: An Illustrated Reference for Successful Cooking.* Des Moines, IA: Meredith Corporation, 1991.

Faas, Patrick. *Around the Roman Table: Food and Feasting in Ancient Rome.* New York: Palgrave Macmillan, 2003.

Hemphill, John and Rosemary. *What Herb Is That? How to Grow and Use the Culinary Herbs.* Mechanicsburg, PA: Stackpole Books, 1990.

Hill, Madalene, and Gwen Barclay. "The Noble Bay," *The Herb Companion.* Retrieved December 15, 2011. http://www.herbcompanion.com/UnCategorized/The-Noble -Bay.aspx.

Leadbetter, Ron. "Apollo," *Encyclopedia Mythica*. Retrieved December 15, 2011. http://www.pantheon.org/articles/a /apollo.html.

Martin, Gary. "Rest on One's Laurels," *The Phrase Finder*. Retrieved December 15, 2011. http://www.phrases.org .uk/meanings/rest-on-his-laurels.html.

McVicar, Jekka. *The Complete Herb Book*. Buffalo, NY: Firefly Books, 2008.

———. *Jekka's Herb Cookbook*. Buffalo, NY: Firefly Books, 2011.

Rombauer, Irma, Marion Rombauer Becker, and Ethan Becker. *Joy of Cooking*. New York: Scribner, 2006.

Tasting Table Chefs' Recipes. "Big Fish: An Aromatic Fish from the River Cottage," *Tasting Table*. Retrieved Dec. 15, 2011. http://www.tastingtable.com/entry_detail /national/3879/An_aromatic_fish_from_the_River _Cottage.htm.

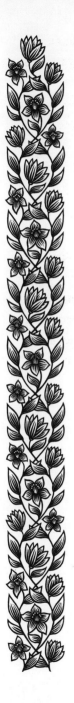

# Herbs for Health and Beauty

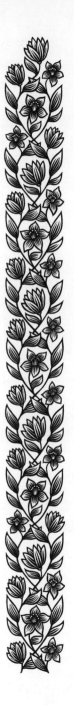

# Herbs for Skin Care

by Cindy Jones, Ph.D.

Growing your own herbs in your gardens to use for skin care purposes can be very rewarding and also bring about significant improvements in the health of your skin.

If you already have herb gardens, you probably have quite a few herbs that can be used for skin care. If you don't already grow herbs, consider growing some of the ones talked about here to use for your skin care.

Skin care is not just for beauty. Skin is an important organ of the body that functions as a barrier to keep water inside the body and other substances outside the body. Resisting infections, regulating body temperature, sensing the environment, communicating nonverbally, and making

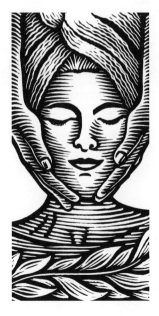

vitamin D are additional roles the skin plays in overall health. Maintaining healthy skin keeps it functioning properly. Herbs also have a beauty of their own, which makes skin care a wonderful way to use them.

Herbs can be used both topically and internally to improve the health of the skin. You may be surprised that common herbs that are grown for culinary purposes can be very important in improving health. Herbs are generally easy to grow and fit into small spaces. Most need very little water and can thrive even without good soil. If you do not have a garden, you can grow many herbs in pots indoors.

## Harvesting and Drying Herbs

Herbs should be cut at their peak. For leafy herbs, harvest before they send out flower stalks. Cut about ½ to ⅔ of the length of the stem, enough to make a bunch about the size of your thumb. Wrap the stems with a rubber band and hang the bunch in a warm, dry space out of direct sunlight to dry. If the herb you are collecting is a flower, pick the flower heads just as they bloom and put them in a basket to dry. Roots should be dug and cleaned in the fall once the plant has died back. Dandelion, however, is an exception, and its root should be dug in the springtime. When herbs are completely dry, store them in glass jars away from direct sunlight.

## Using Herbs Topically

### Teas, Water Infusions, and Decoctions

These watery extracts contain the water-soluble components of the herb and should be used immediately or within 1–2 days if refrigerated.

For a tea, put 1–2 teaspoons dried or fresh herb in a cup or jar. Pour 1 cup very hot, just less than boiling water over the herbs. Steep, covered, for about 5 minutes, and strain.

To make an infusion, steep longer, for 15–30 minutes, before straining. This is basically the same as a tea but stronger.

For a decoction, simmer the herb in water for 30 minutes. A decoction is typically made from woody material such as bark or roots, so it needs the extra time to break down the woody material.

These extracts can be drunk or applied directly to the skin or hair or even used as a gargle.

## Compress

A compress is a way of applying a concentrated herb solution directly to the skin.

Soak a washcloth in an infusion or decoction. Apply the washcloth to the skin and let it sit there.

Common herbs for a compress are chamomile for inflammation or thyme to prevent infection. Oftentimes herb compresses are used in conjunction with massage for relaxation. These herbs might include lavender or clary sage. This is a good way to treat a rash or dermatitis.

## Poultice

A poultice is similar to a compress but uses the whole plant rather than an extract.

Mash or bruise the leaves of an herb. If you are inside, you could use a mortar and pestle. If outside, you could even mash the herb with your teeth if necessary, assuming you are sure it is not toxic if ingested. Apply these herbs directly to the skin. Hold the poultice in place with a gauze bandage.

This method is often used to treat an inflamed, painful part of the body or a wound.

Common herbs for a poultice are mustard poultice on the chest for congestion or sage and chamomile to treat inflammation.

### Infused Oil

An infused oil contains the oil-soluble chemicals of the herb.

Fill a clean quart or pint jar with dried herb (do not use fresh). Cover the herb with a carrier oil such as olive oil, sunflower oil, grapeseed oil, or almond oil. Be sure to push the herb down so it is completely covered with oil.

Let this steep at room temperature for 2 weeks or more, shaking occasionally. Strain out herbs using cheesecloth. Use this oil directly on the skin or in the bath.

### Bath

Use herbs in the bath by putting them in a muslin bag or tying them in a washcloth. Use about ¼ cup herbs per bath.

### Vinegar

Using vinegar is a great way to prepare a mineral-rich extract from herbs.

Mix ½ cup dried or fresh herb with 1 ½ cups cider vinegar. Push the herbs down to make sure they are completely covered with vinegar.

Let this stand for 2–3 weeks in a warm place, shaking frequently. Strain the herbs out using cheesecloth and store in a clean bottle.

When ready to use, dilute the vinegar about 1:10 with clear water.

Use this vinegar as a toner on the face, add to the bath, or use as a hair rinse. Good herbs for a hair rinse are horsetail and sage.

## Tincture

Because it is extracted into alcohol, a tincture is more stable and will last longer than the other extracts.

Fill a pint jar with dried or fresh herb. Cover herb with brandy, vodka, or other alcohol of choice.

Shake daily for 2 weeks. Strain through cheesecloth at this time, or keep as is for use. Store the tincture in a dark glass bottle.

Tinctures are usually taken internally a dropperful at a time, but can also be added to the bath or a tea for topical use.

## Distillates

A distillate, or hydrosol, is the steam collected from heating herbs with water. It contains the volatile molecules of the herb. Distillates are very good for the skin for many reasons and can be used as a toner on the skin, spritzed on for hydration, sprayed to calm a rash or skin irritation, or used as part of a cream or lotion. Home stills are becoming more popular, but you can also purchase a variety of distillates for the skin. We won't go into the how-to here for distilling.

## Steam Inhalation

Steam is a great way to enjoy the benefits of herbs on the skin and in the lungs. Put about ¼ cup dried or fresh herb in a large bowl, and pour boiling water over the herbs. Hold your head over the herbs and inhale the steam. Be careful, though, that the steam does not burn the skin. For added benefit, cover your head with a towel to help hold in the steam. Do this for 1–2 minutes or more.

# Face Care Regimen

A good skin care regimen includes cleansing, toning, and moisturizing. You can incorporate herbs into each phase of this regimen.

## Cleansing

Cleansing removes dirt, debris, makeup, sweat, and excess sebum from the face. Lavender is an herb used historically for cleansing; its name in Latin means "to wash." Other herbs good for cleansing are those that contain saponin, a plant chemical compound that can form a foam. The best known of these herbs is yucca root (*Yucca spp.*), of which there are several species, but others include soapwort (*Saponaria*), licorice (*Glycyrrhiza glabra*), ginseng (*Panax*), yarrow (*Achillea millefolium*), and viola (*Viola*).

Make a decoction of any of these herbs to use as a face wash. Herbs that might be good to mix with a saponin-containing herb include linden, parsley, chamomile, fennel, or lady's mantle.

You might also try purchasing a high-quality melt and pour soap base and add herb extracts to that. Cut up enough melt and pour soap base to make 1 cup. Add about 1 tablespoon infused oil or water infusion, and microwave soap base until melted. Pour this into molds and allow to harden. Remove from mold and it is ready to use.

## Steam Facial

A steam facial can be an occasional addition to your cleansing routine and has an aromatic advantage, too. Any herbs you like can be used. Here is a combination I like:

1 tablespoon chamomile

1 tablespoon rose petals

1 tablespoon fennel leaves

1 tablespoon lavender buds or leaves

Put these herbs in the bottom of a large bowl. Pour boiling water over this and hold your head over the steam for 1–2 minutes. Pat your face dry with a towel.

## Masks

Masks are another addition to cleansing and can have moisturizing benefits as well. Good ingredients for masks include honey, yogurt, ground oatmeal, ground almonds, clay, and ground herbs. You can use a mask about once a week. My favorite mask recipe is as follows, but you can come up with your own combinations too.

### Yogurt Mask

½ cup full fat yogurt (the fat is good for your face but not your arteries!)

2 tablespoons dried or fresh ground herbs (parsley, chamomile, calendula)

Mix together. Apply to face and relax for 10–15 minutes. Wipe clean with a wet washcloth.

## Toning

Toning is done to remove the last traces of cleanser and to restore the natural acid nature of the skin. The skin's normal pH is slightly acidic. This acid mantle of the skin is a protective mechanism to inhibit the growth of bacteria and fungus on the skin. Since vinegar is acidic, it is good to use as a toner;

however, straight vinegar is too strong to use directly on the face, so dilute a vinegar extract about 1:5 or even 1:10 before applying to the face. Herbs used in toners are typically astringent types of herbs. Here is one recipe for an infused vinegar to use as a toner.

*Vinegar Toner*

¼ cup dried cornflowers

¼ cup dried sage

¼ cup dried lady's mantle

1 ½ cups cider vinegar

Place together in a jar, covered, for 2–3 weeks. Strain herbs out and store in a clean bottle. Store the vinegar full strength to prevent bacterial and fungal growth, but dilute vinegar with water, 1 part vinegar to 5 parts water, just before use. If you experience a stinging, then dilute the vinegar more.

Toners are also astringent and tighten the skin. Raspberry leaf is a good astringent herb and can be used as a tea. Make a strong raspberry leaf tea or infusion and apply to the face with a cotton ball.

Tinctures diluted in water about 1:5 can be used as a toner. Try using a tincture made from basil or parsley. Their high vitamin K and vitamin A content will be good for skin. Herbal distillates applied to the face are great toners and hydrators.

### Moisturizing

Only water can add moisture to the skin, but a good moisturizer is typically a mix of water and oil. The water moisturizes and the oil seals the skin to hold in the moisture. Making your own creams can be tricky unless you are a microbiologist or chemist. What you can do, however, is apply a thin film of oil to your face while it is still damp from your toner. Try using an oil infused with calendula; it is rich in vitamin A–related compounds and has good anti-aging properties. Just lightly dab this oil on your face after the toning step.

## Body Care Regimen

Body care is not that much different than face care, but the toning step is usually eliminated, leaving just cleansing and moisturizing.

For cleansing the body, bath herbs are often used. Or if you are a shower person, salt scrubs are quite luxurious. You can put herb mixes for the bath in muslin bags, or more easily just tie them up in a washcloth and put that in your bath water. Good herbs for the bath include oregano, lemon balm, and chamomile. Mix these together in equal amounts.

*Herbal Bath Salts*

> 1 cup Epsom salt
>
> 1 cup table salt
>
> 1 tablespoon baking soda
>
> 1 tablespoon lavender flowers (finely ground in a blender)
>
> 1 tablespoon chamomile flowers
>
> 1 tablespoon rose petals
>
> 1 tablespoon lemon balm leaf

Grind the dried herbs finely in a blender or coffee grinder. It's good to dedicate a coffee grinder to this purpose. Add the finely ground herbs to the other ingredients and mix together.

Add 10 drops lavender essential oil and mix well. Use 2–3 tablespoons or more, if you like, in a bath.

Milk has good moisturizing abilities and is a good addition to an herbal bath. You can add 2 tablespoons of dried milk powder to this recipe as an alternative or leave out the salt and just mix milk powder and herbs. Be creative.

Although it's always good to set aside time in your week for a relaxing herbal bath, for some people it's just not something they do. You can still have a relaxing herbal experience in the shower, though, by using a salt scrub. A salt scrub is gently rubbed on the skin in the shower and then rinsed off. The salt helps to exfoliate and remove the outer dead layer of skin. The oil from the scrub stays behind to moisturize. Be careful, though, because the oil can make the shower stall slippery. You can use salt scrubs on your hands as well to keep them younger looking.

### Herbal Salt Scrub

1 cup oil (olive oil, almond oil, or sunflower oil)

1 cup table salt

1 tablespoon mixed dried herbs of choice
   (chamomile, lavender, rose, linden flower)

Mix all these ingredients together and put in a clean plastic jar for the shower. A more solid oil, like coconut oil or shea butter, can replace half of the oil to make a more solid salt scrub. Just melt the heavier oil in a pan on low heat on the stovetop along with your liquid oil before adding the salt and herbs.

### Massage Oil/Bath Oil

You can add a body oil to the bath water, or apply directly after getting out of the shower, to lock in moisture or as a massage oil. Because all base oils have a different makeup of fatty acids, I like to mix more than one oil so I get more of a variety of fatty acids delivered to my skin. A mixture of olive oil and avocado oil is nice, or olive oil and walnut or sesame oil is also nice. Comfrey infused oil works well in a body oil because it contains allantoin, a substance that helps new skin grow and soothes skin.

### Massage Oil

1 cup olive oil

¼ cup sesame oil

¼ cup comfrey infused oil

¼ cup red clover infused oil

Mix all together and add 10–20 drops essential oil of choice. Put oil in a clean bottle and cap.

### Foot Bath

For someone who spends a lot of time on their feet, a foot bath that contains relaxing herbs as well as antiseptic herbs (to reduce the chance of athlete's foot) can be a wonderful weekly ritual.

¼ cup thyme

¼ cup mint

¼ cup lavender

½ cup hops

Mix dried herbs together and store in a jar. Use about ¼ cup herbs in a muslin bag in a wide tub large enough for your feet. Pour hot water over the herbs and allow to steep until cool enough to put your feet into the water. Put your feet in the tub while you relax.

# Hair Care

Hair is an extension of the skin and can benefit from herbal treatments as well. After shampooing, rinse your hair with an herbal infusion. The herbs you use can help accentuate your hair color. For blond hair use chamomile or calendula, for brunette hair use rosemary, parsley, and sage. Additional herbs to use for hair are those rich in minerals, such as horsetail and red clover.

# Ingesting Herbs for Skin Care

Herbs are rich in vitamins and antioxidants that benefit the skin and reduce the signs of aging. These benefits are just as important (if not more so) when ingested as they are on the surface of the skin. Important vitamins for the skin are vitamins A, C, D, and E. Vitamin C is probably the single most important vitamin for skin care and is involved in making the protein fibers that lay under the skin, giving it support. Herbs that are high in vitamin C include thyme, parsley, basil, and rose hips. Since vitamin C is not stable and diminishes with drying and storage, fresh herbs are best used to get the most benefit in terms of vitamin C content. Use thyme with roasted vegetables, rose hips in tea, parsley in tabbouleh, and basil in pesto.

### Rose Hip Tea

Place 2 tablespoons chopped rose hips in a cup, and pour 1–2 cups boiling water over them. Let this steep for 10–15 minutes. You can sweeten with honey or add peppermint for zing. This makes a lovely tart tea that can be enjoyed hot or cold.

### Tabbouleh

2 cups chopped fresh parsley

1 medium onion, finely chopped

1 small cucumber, chopped

4 medium tomatoes, chopped

1 teaspoon salt

½ teaspoon pepper

½ cup bulgur

5 tablespoons lemon juice

5 tablespoons olive oil

Soak the bulgur ahead of time in water for 1–2 hours to soften. Drain well. Combine all ingredients with bulgur and mix. Serve immediately or chill before serving.

### Pesto

2 cups fresh basil leaves

2 cloves garlic

¾ cup olive oil

3 tablespoons Parmesan cheese

2 tablespoons pine nuts (or walnuts)

Salt and pepper to taste

Put all ingredients in a food processor and pulse until well ground. Use on pasta or bread.

Vitamin A stimulates skin cell regeneration, so it helps healing and diminishes the signs of aging. It also gives skin a healthy color. We all know carrots are high in vitamin A, but so are alfalfa, parsley, dandelions, and violets. Any of these are good added to a leafy salad.

Vitamin K is important in strengthening the capillaries of the skin and in blood clotting. Herbs high in vitamin K include basil, parsley, sage, thyme, coriander, oregano, and marjoram. This sounds like a nice herb mix to use as a multipurpose seasoning. If you take so-called blood-thinning medication such as warfarin, however, then these vitamin K–rich herbs are contraindicated, so talk to your physician first.

## Common Herbs Used in Skin Care

### Calendula

Calendula (*Calendula officinalis*) is also called the pot marigold. It is an annual that grows from seed and readily re-seeds itself. It is a beautiful, bright orange flower that prefers full sun. As an edible flower you can eat it in salads, teas, and rice. Calendula flowers are rich in carotenoids, mucilage, resin, flavonoids, and polysaccharides.

Calendula is best used to stimulate cell growth and promote wound healing. It also has anti-inflammatory, immune-stimulating, antibacterial, and antiviral properties, as well as the ability to promote cell growth, which leads to wound healing. Calendula is best used as an infused oil and is particularly useful for dermatitis and skin issues.

### Chamomile

Although there are two types of chamomile, German chamomile (*Matricaria recutita*) and Roman chamomile (*Chamaemelum nobile*), both are good for skin. They both have a sweet smell and a small daisy-like flower, but German chamomile grows about one foot tall while Roman chamomile grows closer to the ground. They are used on skin for their anti-inflammatory, sedative, antimicrobial, and soothing properties.

The anti-inflammatory activity of chamomile makes it a soothing treatment for skin ailments, particularly eczema, psoriasis, and diaper rash, and it is likewise found in many skin care products. A cup of chamomile tea can help promote sleep and relieve stress. It can also be used as an antiseptic mouthwash.

### Comfrey

Comfrey (*Symphytum officinale*) has been used historically to treat wounds on the skin as well as sprains and broken bones. Use comfrey on wounds as a poultice or an infusion. Comfrey contains allantoin, a chemical that helps skin grow. Comfrey also decreases inflammation. Use teas or infusions of comfrey in the bath. An infused oil of comfrey is nice in a body oil. Once you have comfrey growing, you will likely always have it growing, as it is very easy to grow and reproduces rapidly.

### Fennel

Fennel (*Foeniculum vulgare*) grows best in good soil and full sun. It can grow to four feet or even higher and readily resows itself. Fennel is typically used as a culinary herb and can aid digestion. For the skin it can be used for deep cleansing and in a steam facial. It can help soften fine lines in aging skin. It is soothing and anti-inflammatory. Use crushed fennel seeds in tea bags on the eyes to reduce swelling.

### Lavender

Lavender (*Lavandula angustifolia*) is a small shrub that grows best in lime soil and full sun. It is one of the most prized cosmetic herbs, with a scent that some find intoxicating. In Latin its name means "to wash," and it has been used in soaps and cosmetics for ages. It is great to use in a steam facial, as the scent can also promote relaxation. Its antiseptic properties make it a good choice to use on damaged skin such as acne, wounds, burns, and scratches. Use it in an infused oil or a tea on the skin.

## Lemon Balm

Lemon balm (*Melissa officinalis*) is a member of the mint family and typically grows quite well in both sun and shade. European settlers in the United States brought lemon balm with them for its anti-anxiety properties to lift their spirits. Lemon balm has a mild sedative effect and makes a great addition to tea blends for drinking. It can also lessen the sting of insect bites. Medical studies show it has antiviral and antibacterial properties, and it is a common addition to lip balms to prevent the development of cold sores. Lemon balm is nice to use in a bath to promote relaxation and relieve the sting of sunburn.

## Red Clover

Red clover (*Trifolium pratense*) is a member of the legume family, so it can be used to improve your garden soil. The flower heads are rich in phytoestrogens, which help to "plump" and soften the skin and keep it young looking. Red clover is very useful for chronic skin conditions like eczema and psoriasis. It is also good to drink as a tea. I like using red clover in a body and massage oil to provide phytoestrogens.

## Rose

Rose (*Rosa spp.*), the Queen of Herbs, comes in many different species, all of which are good for skin. Because there are many different types, make sure you find a variety that grows well in your soil type; ask at a reputable garden center. Rose petals can help soften skin and are useful in a toner as an astringent skin hydrator. The seed heads of rose, the rose hips, are rich in vitamins A, B, C, E, and K and can be used to make a tea. Because of rose's aroma and ability to reduce anxiety, I like to use it in a steam facial.

## Sage

Sage (*Salvia officinalis*) grows well with little water and in poor soil. Most people use sage as a culinary herb, but its use as a culinary herb to season meats and stuffing most likely came about because of its antimicrobial properties, which decrease the likelihood of spoilage. Sage's antimicrobial properties also make it useful to decrease the risk of skin infection from cuts and scrapes. Add sage to your bath water, or use a tea as a gargle for treating gingivitis, sore gums, and bad breath. Because it has a tendency to dry mucous membranes, sage can be used in steam for a runny nose.

## Thyme

Thyme (*Thymus vulgaris*) prefers full sun and well-drained soil. Since there are over 300 varieties of thyme, you are sure to find one you will like. Most grow low and can be used as ground covers. Thyme is a great culinary herb that goes especially well with mushrooms. It has strong antimicrobial properties, so it can be used to treat mouth infections and protect cuts and scrapes on the skin from becoming infected. It is analgesic, making it a good herb to use in a foot soak to promote relaxation and prevent athlete's foot.

# Flowers for Chemo

### ❧ by Lisa Mc Sherry ❧

Having cancer is like no other experience and is a remarkably unique journey. Based on personal experience, there are a number of herbs (including flower essences and essential oils) that support a person going through a cancer regimen.

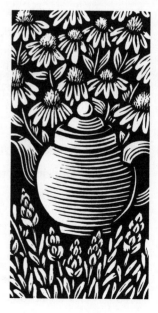

The idea for this article came as I was struggling with my own cancer experience. In late 2009, just before my forty-third birthday, I was diagnosed with breast cancer. After fumbling through a bewildering maze of information and options, I chose surgery and chemotherapy, followed by a five-year regimen of tamoxifen to prevent a recurrence. The entire odyssey was stressful, and no matter how well I thought I was doing, there were times when the only thing to do was have a good cry. Having cancer didn't hurt, but surgery was taxing and chemotherapy completely redefined my idea of what constitutes "healthy." I am not a doctor nor a medical professional, but perhaps what I learned along the way will be of use to you if you ever find yourself on the same journey.

Cancer results from the uncontrolled growth of abnormal cells, which form tumors. Blood flow is redirected to the tumors and away from healthy cells nearby. Moreover, cancer cells can travel elsewhere in the body and produce additional tumors (so breast cancer cells can be found in the liver or lungs), spreading the destruction. The tumors will eventually overwhelm the organ or tissue where they are located.

Many herbal therapies use the natural pharmaceutical properties to restore or support the body's immune system. At this time there are no herbs proven to cure cancer. Moreover, "natural" does not always mean "safe," and everything you do, including "just" taking vitamins, needs to be done with the knowledge and under the supervision of your health care provider. If there is a common agreement on a dosage, I've provided it; otherwise, consult with your herbalist or naturopath as to the best dosage for your situation.

## Surgery Support

Providing support for the body in preparation for surgery is a wise idea, and ideally is started three or four weeks prior to the surgery date. If you don't have that kind of time, start as soon as you can; any support is better than none. Eat a nutritious diet low in fat and high in protein and vitamins. High-quality protein, such as that found in fish, poultry, nuts, and seeds, is crucial because protein is required for tissue healing.

Some of the most important surgery supplements are antioxidants: vitamins A and C, selenium, and zinc. These nutrients can help reduce tissue damage after surgery. Anthocyanidins, which are potent antioxidants in deep red and blue fruits, are excellent to add to your diet. Immune-building herbs such as echinacea (*Echinacea spp.*) also help ready the system for surgery (5–20 ml tincture). Tonic and strengthening herbs such as Siberian ginseng (*Eleutherococcus senticosus*, 5–10 ml), gentian (*Gentiana lutea*), and astragalus (*Astragalus membranaceus*, 15 ml) can help with stress, digestion, and immune function. Horsetail (*Equisetum arvense*) will support wound healing because the herb is high in silica, which can help strengthen tissues. Goldenseal root (*Hydrastis canadensis*) works as a tonic and is a natural, mild infection fighter. Herbs that can thin the blood, such as ginkgo (*Ginkgo biloba*, 40–160 mg), red clover (*Trifolium pratense*), and alfalfa (*Medicago sativa*) should not be taken before surgery.

Post-surgery, (decaffeinated) teas can be very helpful in reducing the side effects of anesthesia and pain-relieving drugs; they are also comforting in the absolutely unpleasant environment of the hospital. Teas that include ginger (*Zingiber officinale*, 250–1000 mg) will help reduce nausea and that woozy feeling that lingers. Vitamin C promotes wound healing, and 500–2000 mg of bromelain, an enzyme derived from pineapple, can reduce postsurgical inflammation and may help with digestion.

If you want to help speed healing and minimize the appearance of scars, the two best essential oils to use are lavender and helichrysum. A simple recipe is to combine ¼ teaspoon vitamin E oil, 3 teaspoons aloe vera gel or juice, and 3 drops pure lavender or helichrysum essential oil. Blend well and apply several times a day. In my case, a friend sent me a jar of comfrey salve that was a miracle, minimizing the scars and speeding the healing. All of my surgeons were impressed with how quickly and well I healed.

## Radiation Support

Radiation is a common therapeutic complement to surgery, or it may be used alone to treat the cancer. Radiation is targeted to a specific tumor or group of cancer cells; it penetrates them and activates the process of programmed cell death. It damages cellular DNA in all cells, healthy and cancerous. Side effects of radiation include anemia, fatigue, nausea, diarrhea, hair loss, skin irritation or burns, and sterility.

Kelp (*Laminaria*) is very high in iodine, which helps regulate the thyroid, helping it process out the radiation. Start taking kelp with the first diagnosis and keep going right through radiotherapy treatment and for months afterward. If using an extract, the dosage is 15 drops, 4 doses per day in water. Yarrow (*Achillea millefolium*) is a nervous system and circulatory tonic and should be taken for the duration of the treatment. Infuse 1 tablespoon yarrow in 8 ounces hot water, covered, for 20 minutes. Sip 1 teaspoon as needed every 20 minutes.

Spirulina (*Arthrospira*), a type of algae, contains the highest plant source of gamma-linolenic acid (GLA), a fatty acid that strengthens immunity and inhibits excessive cell division. Spirulina can be added to juice or smoothies or taken in capsule form. Ginger can help reduce stomach cramps, nausea, and vomiting. It is also a natural antioxidant and anti-inflammatory and helps prevent ulcers from developing by protecting the lining of the stomach. It is best taken fresh or as an herbal tea, but can also be added to food.

# Chemotherapy Support

Chemotherapy (chemo) may be used before, during, or after radiation and surgery. Chemo involves giving the patient chemicals (orally or intravenously) that circulate throughout the body and are toxic to cells. Chemo halts cell reproduction and growth, especially in rapidly dividing cells, and cancer cells are the most rapidly dividing in the body. There are more than forty different drugs used in chemo, and most patients will receive a mixture of several in an individualized cocktail. All of the filtering organs are negatively affected and need support. The most common side effects of chemo are nausea, hair loss, mouth sores, constipation or diarrhea, fatigue, weakness, taste impairment, loss of appetite, low blood count, infection, neuropathy, joint pain, and difficulty sleeping.

Aloe vera contains a water-soluble compound called acemannan, which is a potent immune stimulant and antitumor agent. Therapeutic dosing has not been established, but a guideline would be 30 ml, 3 times a day. Drinking 4 fluid ounces of aloe vera juice (on an empty stomach) can be helpful in soothing the intestinal tract. Chronic use of aloe can lead to potassium deficiency, especially when used with licorice, thiazide diuretics, and steroids.

Astralagus helps restore white blood cells, so it is beneficial after chemotherapy, which tends to depress those counts to subpar levels. Traditional Chinese medicine uses this herb for night sweats, fatigue, loss of appetite, weakness, and diarrhea, all of which are possible side effects of chemotherapy. Chamomile (*Matricaria chamomilla*) supports the balance of the digestive system and the parasympathetic nervous system. It helps balance the metabolism to recover more quickly after shock and allows the appetite and vitality to return more readily after each chemo session.

Milk thistle (*Silybum marianum*) is a major liver tonic but is *not* recommended if your cancer was hormone positive. This plant enhances liver detoxification and supports the growth of healthy liver cells. It contains a bioflavonoid known as silymarin, one constituent of which is silibinin. For liver disease, 400–1000 mg is the recommended dosage. Alfalfa (*Medicago sativa*) supports the digestive system in general. Rose hips offer support to the kidney, liver, and adrenals in particular and are an antioxidant and a high source of iron and vitamin C.

Parsley (*Petroselinum hortense*) offers powerful support for those whose vitality has been severely compromised. Chopped and mixed into a white sauce or eaten with a bit of fish or salad, parsley is a useful source of iron, minerals, and vitamin C. Fennel (*Foeniculum vulgare*) is a metabolic tonic especially directed to the health and function of the pancreas. Ginger is a metabolic tonic that enlivens the digestion and the metabolism in general and is therefore helpful in speeding the return to normal functioning after toxic shock.

Licorice (*Glycyrrhiza glabra*) assists in the recovery from severe adrenal shock. The adrenal glands are depleted catastrophically when a toxic shock is administered to our systems without warning, as in the case of all treatments administered directly into the bloodstream. The dosage for licorice in a tincture is 3–10 ml. Eating less fat can help with diarrhea, and probiotics will help balance the intestines. Shark oil can counterbalance anemia when 1000 mg are taken 3–6 times daily.

# Other Issues

When I lost my hair, I kept my scalp healthy through weekly exfoliating with a washcloth and judicious use of moisturizer (the same stuff I use on my face, nothing fancy). When the hair began to regrow (about six weeks after the last treatment), I began using Sea Chi scalp treatment product. (Detailed product information is given at the end of this article.) My hair grew back very quickly, again amazing everyone around me. Throughout the entire odyssey I used the essential oil product Sleep, A Bedtime Ritual to help me sleep.

Cancer's odyssey brings with it overwhelming amounts of anger, anxiety, and fear, all beginning with those terrible words "You have cancer." It is not confined to the patient, but encompasses everyone in his or her life; sometimes it can be much more difficult to watch your loved ones struggle while you stand by helplessly, supportive but impotent. For all of you, aromatherapy can be an excellent program. Scents like neroli, chamomile, and lavender are relaxing and antidepressant. You don't need to do anything elaborate. I put a few drops of oil on a couple of handkerchiefs, and carried them with me or tucked them into my pillowcase at night. A more elegant solution is to purchase an aromatherapy necklace and extra scent pads. Mine is a small pewter locket decorated with the Celtic spiral of life; it opens and small pads can be placed inside. As the locket warms from being against my skin, the scent is gently released.

When you emerge from the cancer process, you are likely to feel run down and exhausted, perhaps even toxic. When you feel ready (and probably no sooner than three months post-chemo), consider doing a very gentle liver detox. A course of liver-supportive herbs such as milk thistle, burdock (*Arctium lappa*), and shiitake (*Lentinula edodes*) is a good way to go. Green and white teas offer phytochemicals that suppress cancer cell reproduction and block enzymes needed for tumor invasion; they also help collect fat-soluble toxins into the bowels for elimination. Drinking 4–8 cups of high-quality tea each day is the recommended dosage, although using dietary supplements will do just as well.

Many of us have experienced profound changes to our body, leading to strong feelings of unease and psychic distress. A product I have found valuable in helping me reintegrate and re-map my body is Blue Morpho Body Oil.

There are a number of Bach flower essences you may be drawn to work with during this time. Crab apple cleanses poisons; gentian, gorse, and mimulus assist when you are grappling with doubt; hornbeam helps when you are feeling overburdened; oak assists when fighting against overwhelming odds; olive eases suffering; rock rose rescues in cases where there is no hope; and star of Bethlehem is perfect for mitigating the stress of shock. I also found willow useful in accepting what I couldn't change.

How you navigate your way through the cancer odyssey will be unique to you, your needs, your situation, and your support. I hope these plants are your allies if you ever find yourself on this journey.

## Products I Recommend

Blue Morpho Body Oil from *Kate's Magik*, http://www.kates magik.com/blue-morpho.html. Also available at *Isabella*, http://www.isabellacatalog.com/p/Blue-Morpho-Body -Oil.cfm.

Sleep, A Bedtime Ritual from *Essence of Vali*, http://essence
ofvali.com/products-page/natural-sleep-aids/sleep-a
-bedtime-ritual. Also available through *Isabella*, http://
www.isabellacatalog.com/p/Sleep-Aromatherapy.cfm.

Sea Chi Leave On Moisturizing Treatment & Hair Growth
Formula from *Sea Chi*, http://www.seachi.com/leave
-moisturizing-treatment-hair-growth-formula-8oz240ml
-p-44.html. Also available through *Isabella*, http://www
.isabellacatalog.com/p/Sea-Chi-Organics-Leave-On
-Moisturizing-Treatment-Hair-Growth-Formula.cfm.

Aromatherapy necklace. Several sources and styles. Mine is
from Nature's Alchemy at *Vitacost.com*, http://www
.vitacost.com/productResults.aspx?x=0&y=0&ntk
=products&ss=1&Ntt=aromatherapy%20necklace.

Bach Flower Remedies, http://bachflower.com.

# Sources

Alschuler, Lise, and Karolyn Gazella. *The Definitive Guide to
Cancer: An Integrative Approach to Prevention, Treatment,
and Healing.* Third edition. Berkeley, CA: Celestial Arts,
2010. Strongly recommended reading.

Balch, Phyllis A, CNC. *Prescription for Nutritional Healing.*
Fourth edition. New York: Avery, 2006.

Boston Women's Health Book Collective. *Our Bodies, Ourselves.*
New York: Touchstone, 1996.

*The Herb Companion*, http://www.herbcompanion.com.

Leaf, Fern, BA, NE, NC, NANP. "Nutritional Support During Radiation and Chemotherapy Treatments." *Nutrition*

# Hyssop: Nature's Medicinal Storeroom

### ⤜ by Susan Pesznecker ⤛

Have you worked much with hyssop? It's a wonderful herb and one that I use regularly in my garden and my own herbal practices. Hyssop (pronounced *HIH-supp*) is easy to grow, yielding a beautiful, fragrant plant with long-lasting spears of flowers that attract bees and butterflies. A member of the mint family, hyssop has a wide range of medicinal uses and is particularly good for winter colds and flu as well as being a potent immune stimulant. Hyssop also makes a fragrant, delicious tea.

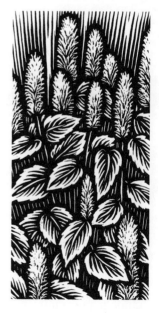

*Hyssopus officinalis* is a semi-evergreen shrub that grows to two feet, producing narrow, dark green leaves and sprays of blue or bluish purple double-lipped flowers that appear in June or July and last into the autumn months. (Occasionally, the plants may have white or reddish flowers.) Hyssop is native to southern Europe, where it grows wild. Thankfully for the rest of us, it's also easy to cultivate by seed or cutting in temperate climates around the world.

When grown in the garden, hyssop prefers dry, well-drained soil and lots of sun. Once it begins growing vigorously, it benefits—as most herbs do—from regular and rather aggressive clipping, to which it responds by growing even more robust and bushy. It's a beautiful and useful garden plant, its deep green foliage contrasting with the brilliant floral spears, and it attracts birds, bees, and butterflies to the garden. Some reports also note its value in discouraging certain garden pests, like the cabbage white butterfly.

Hyssop is a brilliant healing herb as well. The *officinalis* in hyssop's scientific name stems from the Latin word *officina*, meaning "office" or "storeroom." In medieval times, much of what was known about herbs and herbal workings was preserved by monks, with herbal apothecaries operating out of monastic storerooms. These storerooms would, over centuries, morph into our modern pharmacies. The use of *officinalis* is a reference to these times and, when included in the scientific name, points to a plant's value as a medicinal herb. And indeed, hyssop has a wide range of uses in medicinal herbalism. In ancient times, it was regarded as a general use herb that could treat or cure almost anything.

Hyssop is a member of the family Lamiaceae, the flowering herb family known collectively as "mints." Hyssop's cousins include peppermint, thyme, lemon balm, and a number of other deeply fragrant plants. Today we know that hyssop's active constituents include volatile oils (responsible for hyssop's ethereal scent), terpenes, flavonoids, and tannins. Volatile oils tend to be antiseptic and anti-inflammatory, and many—including the camphor found in hyssop—help dilate the bronchial tree, easing breathing. The terpene *marrubiin* is known to be a strong expectorant, meaning it helps one cough up and clear phlegm from the lungs. Flavonoids are antioxidant compounds that maintain cell health and slow age-related changes in cells, tissues, and blood vessels, while tannins are astringent in nature and known for staunching blood flow and treating infections.

Topically, hyssop infusions are both cleansing and stimulating, making them good for treating circulatory problems, infections, and fatigued muscles and joints. A poultice may be applied to treat aching joints as well as bruises and small wounds. The antiseptic volatile oils in hyssop make the infusions useful in treating simple wounds and wound infections. A strong hyssop infusion also makes a relaxing, restorative bath. Adding a few drops of hyssop essential oil to ¼ cup carrier oil—such as apricot or sunflower—creates a massage oil that can relieve joint pain and, when rubbed on the chest, ease breathing problems associated with asthma or respiratory illness. Adding a bit of eucalyptus, rosemary, and/or thyme oil creates a "vapor rub" that may be even more effective than the plain mixture.

*Safety note:* Hyssop's undiluted essential oil is used by some herbalists to treat various conditions; however, it is extremely strong and has been known to induce seizures in some people. Therefore, it should only be used in its concentrated form by professionals. Some countries actually restrict the use and sale of hyssop essential oil. Hyssop in any form should not be used by pregnant women, as it may stimulate uterine contractions.

Taken orally, a hyssop infusion promotes calm and relaxation and has gently sedative properties. It aids treatment of lung infections by opening the airways, stimulating mucus formation, and stimulating expectoration. Hippocrates mentioned hyssop to treat pleurisy and lung congestion, and both Dioscorides and Galen likewise recorded its use for asthma and a number of other respiratory conditions. As with many members of the mint family, hyssop also soothes and relaxes the gastrointestinal tract, making it valuable in treating indigestion, gas, and colic. It may ease the pain of sore throat and tonsillitis. In recent years, hyssop has shown potential benefits as an immune stimulant and antiviral agent; it is being investigated for supportive treatment in those infected with the herpes virus and the human immunodeficiency virus (HIV).

In addition to its medicinal value, hyssop has a number of unique and interesting uses. Its name translates with almost no change from the ancient Greek, and hyssop is mentioned in the Christian Bible (which identifies it as an herb used in cleansing holy places) and in the works and writings of many ancient and medieval herbalists, including Hippocrates, Dioscorides, and Galen. From the ancient Greeks to medieval folk practitioners, hyssop was regarded as an ideal herb for purification, protection, and cleansing. It was hung in bunches as protection against the evil eye and burned in living spaces as a smudge to clear away dangerous spirits and purify the surrounds. These practices continue today; hyssop infusion is frequently used in Catholic ceremony to fill the aspergillum, a ritual tool used for asperging and purifying with holy water.

The ancient Romans also used hyssop to make a fragrant and intoxicating wine. In modern times, hyssop leaves provide color for the alcoholic beverage known as absinthe and are a key part of the liqueur known as Chartreuse, a French beverage composed of more than 130 herbal extracts. Like many members of the Laminaceae family, hyssop is also used frequently in perfumery.

Medieval folks used hyssop in cooking, where it was one of a mixture of herbs that helped "preserve" meats. In reality, the herbs probably weren't much help in actually preserving the meat, but likely helped mask the scent of slow spoilage. People today don't cook much with hyssop, finding it to be too strong to be palatable in everyday foods. However, as mentioned earlier, it makes a delicious tea. Steep 1 teaspoon dried herb or 2 teaspoons fresh crushed herb in 1 cup freshly boiled water for about 5 minutes. Sweeten if desired with a bit of sugar, honey, or agave syrup. This pure infusion—herbalists refer to a one-herb mixture as a "simple"—is heavenly all by itself. It also blends well with other herbs and spices.

You can start hyssop in the garden from seeds once the ground warms. Germination is slow, however, and you may have better luck starting seeds early indoors and then transplanting the young plants. Keep the soil barely damp until the plants begin to grow vigorously; after that, hyssop benefits from slightly dry soil and regular feeding with an all-purpose plant food. Hyssop will reward you with gorgeous flowers and foliage—it makes a nice mid-height plant in an herb garden and is lovely against a fence or backdrop.

To harvest, snip hyssop's aerial parts during the summer as the plant flowers. Remember, the flowers are beloved by bees and butterflies, so be sure to leave some for them as well. Dry the cuttings in a warm room out of direct sunlight, and store in glass jars in a light-tight cupboard for up to two years.

## Sources

Skinner, Monica. "Companion Gardening—Compatible Plants." *ICanGarden.com*. May 28, 2008. http://www .icangarden.com/document.cfm?task=viewdetail&item id=7198.

Wolters Kluwer Health. "Hyssop." *Drugs.com*. 2009. http:// www.drugs.com/npp/hyssop.html.

# Calming Down: Herbal and Natural Remedies for Stress and Anxiety

### ⁂ by Sally Cragin ⁂

In the 1970s it was "mellow out," and in the '90s it was "take a chill pill," but whatever decade it is, we always have some mindset that urges others to *stop being so upset!* Stress and anxiety have become twin polestars and are likened to be the root cause of many medical and psychological disorders.

So…are they? And if so, what can you do about it—especially if you don't want to enter the world of pharmacopeia? (Remember the Rolling Stones' song "Mother's Little Helper"?) First, start reading. A couple of years ago I wrote a piece for the *Herbal Almanac* on herbs that help give you energy. I had just given birth to my second child and was avoiding

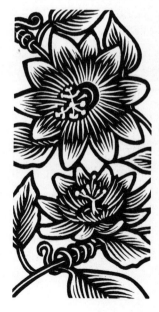

caffeinated coffee. How's that for crazy! But after the economic recession hit in 2008, I found that a lot of clients who came to me for astrological consultations were nervous and upset. If they had a job they hated, they were afraid to leave it. If they had lost a job, they were afraid they'd never find another. In short, numerous people suffered from stress and anxiety to a degree I'd never seen before in two decades of talking to clients.

My comments to them were always along the lines of: "If the stress and anxiety you're feeling seem insurmountable, you definitely should talk to a medical professional. However, there are some natural palliatives you can use to treat stress and anxiety. And yes, chamomile tea is one of them. You can also look at avoiding substances that stimulate you, such as caffeine, chocolate, nicotine, and refined sugars." I'd also advise them to see whether they weren't just hungry, as feeling blah or stressed-out is sometimes connected to low blood sugar. Here's an easy fix for that: slices of apple with peanut butter. Or just a banana. Getting simple sugars and protein in your system will make you feel more energetic.

But there were so many clients in such a state of anxiety that I got curious about the realm of stress-easing substances, and I found there are a lot of palliatives available.

## Herbs and Elixirs

Let's start alphabetically. Ashwagandha, or *Withania somnifera*, comes in a variety of forms. This shrub is from India and prefers tropical climates. The root is used as a remedy, and its main ingredients are steroidal alkaloids and steroidal lactones. In 2009, a variety of professionals from the Canadian College of Naturopathic Medicine at the University of Toronto and

McMaster University conducted research on members of the Canadian Union of Postal Workers using this herb along with traditional psychotherapy. They found that "naturopathic treatment including *Withania somnifera*, a multivitamin, dietary counseling and cognitive-behavioral therapy appears to be a safe and effective, with benefit over standardized psychotherapy in the treatment of mild to severe generalized anxiety in the Canada Post worker population."[1]

Visiting other cultures (even if one can only do this through research) is an entertaining way to learn about different substances, and it turns out that India abounds with various ingredients designed to help you find your inner "om." Chyavanprash is a remedy comprising more than three dozen herbs, but it is considered an individual treatment. The primary ingredient is Indian gooseberry, which is rich in vitamin C and is said to have anti-aging properties and to promote health, particularly to hair and eyes.[2]

Let's cross an ocean and visit Polynesia. There you'll find natives imbibing a native berry called kava (*Piper methysticum*). This is said to have relaxing effects and has been used for anti-anxiety. You can purchase this at some health food stores and on the Internet (where everything can be found, if you know what you're looking for!). I've used kava-kava every few months, particularly if I'm feeling overwhelmed or if I've dealt with one difficult person too many. I've found it tremendously effective at taking off any potential "edge" I might feel, but I'm also mindful that the U.S. Food and Drug Administration (FDA) issued an advisory about the possible side effects and risks associated with prolonged and repeated ingestion of kava, including liver damage.

At various times I've also been in environments where people smoke or where smokers are present. I've found that the secondhand smoke is annoying and stressful, and research continues on the effects of secondhand smoke. But consider this: had Christopher Columbus headed west and landed on Bora Bora instead of the Canary Islands, we would have had centuries of ingesting Kava Kocktails instead of passing that pipe of peace.

Back in Europe, valerian[3] has been known to assist with anxiety, digestion, and sleep disorders since the era of Hippocrates, who referenced valerian for a variety of ills. Later, Galen (second century CE) recommended valerian for sleep disorders. In the Elizabethan period, valerian was used for its calming effects, on nervous disorders including heart palpitations. As recently as World War II, valerian was given to help counteract the stress brought on by air raids.

Over-the-counter commercial preparations of valerian usually comprise the root or parts of the plant material. It can come in a tea or as capsules. I have found valerian to be useful when first taken, but if I take it more than a few days at a time, it seems to lose its efficacy. Valerian is highly aromatic, but not in a floral, daub-behind-your-ears way.

Passionflower (*Passiflora incarnata*)[4] is another plant that can be found in the Americas as well as Europe. Traditional uses include treatment for stress and sleeplessness. I've found passionflower turning up in various natural food stores more and more. It's an herbal tea ingredient or a capsule (the plant, flower, and leaves are powdered). I don't like it as a hot tea, because of the tanginess, but it's a delicious iced tea brew. Just steep two bags of passionflower and two bags of peppermint tea in a quart of hot water and let cool.

I've read varying recommendations on dosages of passionflower, and the accepted wisdom seems to be that you can drink one to four cups of tea for anxiety or sleeplessness. Personally I've had no reactions to this plant—it's a benign and aromatic addition to the cornucopia of stress-relieving herbs!

Even more fragrant is licorice root (*Glycyrrhiza glabra*). It's commonly grown in Mediterranean countries, the Near East, and Asia, as well as the East Coast and prairie states in the United States. Licorice is considered a food rather than a drug by our Food and Drug Administration. One study showed that a form of licorice extract (not available in the U.S.) had beneficial effects against hepatitis C in clinical trials.[5]

Licorice root was used by native Americans for toothache, and in Chinese medicine it's considered to have detoxifying effects and is widely used. Be warned, however, that ingesting wild licorice can raise blood pressure.

Licorice is a plant I've seldom seen in the wild, but not for want of looking. Usually, if I'm out in the woods, I bring one of my favorite books, the *Peterson Field Guide to Medicinal Plants*, which has photographs as well as illustrations of common forest and field plants. One of the few plants listed that is considered to have been used traditionally for restlessness and anxiety is figwort (*Scrophularia marilandica*). This grows on the East Coast and in the Gulf states and the northern prairie states, but in all my field trips I've never seen it.

When you read books that describe traditional uses for herbs, you'll find many plants that were used for toothache, wound care, bronchial ailments, and indigestion—typical ailments of a pre-modern era. Very few address psychological or emotional states of mind, except for cannabis, of course, which is also prescribed for nausea, and is now (famously) legal for prescription purposes in parts of Europe and sixteen U.S. states (as of fall 2011).[6]

## Pressure Points for Stress Relief

If you're by yourself, you can relieve stress by gently massaging the point on your wrist below the pinky side of your hand.[7] Rub in a circle without pinching. Another good spot is what's called the "third eye"—between the eyebrows. A gentle circular rubbing motion should help relieve stress; try not to pinch or rub too quickly. Another place on the body is the "crooked marsh," which is on the inside of your arm. Bend your elbow, and below the crease there is a sensitive spot. Another location on the arm is the "inner gate," which is two and a half finger-widths from your wrist crease.

When I was testing the efficacy of this method of stress relief, I found it helpful to put a dot with a marker on the points on my hands and arms to remind me during the day to do this small massage. I didn't feel a vast sense of relief, but when I was sampling all these products and practices, I wasn't in a particularly high state of anxiety—no matter how close the deadline got!

You'll definitely need a partner to help with some spots. I contorted myself to reach the "heavenly pillar," which is the back of the head, one finger-width below the base of your skull. You're supposed to massage the ropy muscles on either side of your spine, but it would have been easier with another set of hands.

# Smells and Bells

I enjoy experimenting with aromatherapeutic methods, as they are generally quick and easy. I find I have no need of the violet-leaf extract or the valerian tincture, but I do crave citrus and spicy smells. The oils I enjoy include peppermint, lime, rosemary, geranium, sandlewood, and lavender. Grapefruit and peppermint (in a 2:1 ratio) make for a refreshing scent—fresh and invigorating. Lavender is pleasant in a sleeping pillow and is the herb most frequently mentioned as a "stress reliever." You can imbibe it by anointing your skin with the oil (a mixed-down version, not the essential kind) or by wrapping lavender blossoms in a cambric handkerchief. Sandalwood is so rare and expensive, I use it sparingly. Having a small wooden box in a dark corner, with some clean glass vials and some droppers, is an entertaining diversion. It's hard to stay stressed-out when you're uncapping bottles and inhaling intensely satisfying fragrances.

## Final Thoughts and an Astrological Perspective

Stress is a symptom, not a cause. If you can figure out what's getting you stressed (traffic, encounters with difficult people, lack of time to do a job the best you can), then you may be able to anticipate similar circumstances recurring. In my work as an astrologer, I find that people who enjoy high-stress situations often have a natal full moon (when they were born, the moon was full). Therefore, they seek out environments that are at a high rev. Anything less than 90 miles per hour bores them silly. However, some clients get overwhelmed by small events. These folks often are the ones who were born when the moon was waning or new.

If you find that your anxiety follows a pattern, or that you do get exceptionally stressed-out when the moon is full, you should keep track of the lunar cycles and mark them in red in your personal calendar. And when the lunar phases coincide with menstrual patterns, you ladies can always tell yourself, "Well, I'm in tune with the moon!"

## Notes

1. Kieran Cooley, Orest Szczurko, Dan Perri, Edward J. Mills, Bob Bernhardt, Qi Zhou, and Dugald Seely, "Naturopathic Care for Anxiety," PLoS One, August 31, 2009, http://www.ncbi.nlm.nih.gov/pmc/articles/PMC 2729375/?tool=pmcentrez.

2. Dr. Deepa Apte, "Chyawanprash: The Ultimate Natural Health Supplement," NaturalHealthWeb.com, http://www.naturalhealthweb.com/articles/DeepaApte1.html.

3. The Office of Dietary Supplements, "Valerian," National Institutes of Health, reviewed January 16, 2008, http://ods.od.nih.gov/factsheets/valerian.

4. "Passionflower," University of Maryland Medical Center, reviewed June 23, 2011, http://www.umm.edu/altmed/articles/passionflower-000267.htm.

5. National Center for Complementary and Alternative Medicine, "Licorice Root," National Institutes of Health, http://nccam.nih.gov/health/licoriceroot.

6. "16 Legal Medical Marijuana States and DC," ProCon.org, http://medicalmarijuana.procon.org/view.resource.php?resourceID=000881.

7. "Acupressure Points for Relieving Anxiety and Nervousness," HerbShop.com, http://www.herbalshop.com/Acupressure/Acupressure_20.html.

# Herbalism and
# Energetic Healing

### ⤜ by Calantirniel ⤛

It is said herbal medicine is the oldest system for healing ourselves in
existence. The origins can be traced
back to stone-age humans many thousands of years ago. Whether this came
about through trial and error, observing animals, or being connected to
nature, historical records reveal a vast
and diverse amount of plant healing
information that is still relevant and
usable today.

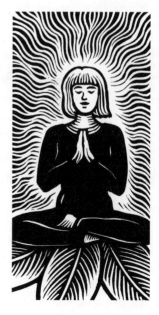

Now, with awareness of the possible dangers of human-created chemical
prescription and/or over-the-counter
drugs, which include serious systemic
injury and even death, people find
themselves seeking the comfort of a
well-documented and historically relevant form of healing through fungi and

plants—the very best natural chemists, both having been around much longer than we have!

The drawbacks of applying herbal medicine, while not many, are worthy of study. A particular problem with using natural diet and herbs for healing is timing. Between the implementation of herbal therapies and the desired results, many uncomfortable cleansing reactions can surface that may even be painful for the client, and the time needed for the herbal therapies to work properly can cause more pain than the client wishes to struggle with.

While it is ideal to treat an herbal client in the early stages of disease, we do not live in an ideal world. Clients often come to us as a last resort, after many years of taking suppressive medicines that removed painful symptoms instantly but only temporarily. Unfortunately, not only has the core issue remained unaddressed, but the residues of these chemicals have not been eliminated because of their unnatural chemical structures. They accumulate in the client's system, rendering the drug ineffective as well as causing side effects, and that is when another suppressive drug is then recommended. When a perceived undesired action in the body is suppressed through sheer external chemical force, the body will attempt to find ways that relieve this suppression, and it often does so by causing a new problem, which is viewed as yet another thing to suppress. Over time, there are many problems to address, not just the original condition. It's no wonder it can take herbs a long time to work in these cases!

While usually inexpensive, herbal therapies can be not only time-consuming but also quite laborious to administer. If you're ill, it can be too much work to do yourself, so it's good to get a family member or friend to help. If hiring a health professional (like an at-home nurse) to administer, double-check with the laws of your area to see if this is possible.

The detoxifying portion of herbal therapies can have other undesired effects, such as cravings for all the unhealthy things the patient finds addicting—and likely all the unhealthy habits that assisted in bringing about the serious chronic illness. And while herbs can address the detoxifying and nutritional needs to move the body toward healing, they cannot correct the origin of the disease imprint that is the deeper reason for nearly any health condition. This usually happens during a traumatic event and is often forgotten. The trauma could have even happened to others in the family, which can make the imprint appear to be hereditary.

So how can herbalists shorten the time needed for herbal protocol and also lessen pain and cravings, thereby facilitating healing as quickly and comfortably as physically possible? We can integrate non-invasive and yet effective techniques that even conventional medicine currently uses with a measurable level of success: energy medicine.

## Combining Herbalism and Energy Medicine

Energy medicine is also called vibrational medicine or energetic healing. There is a large variety of methods available, ranging from more popular systems like Reiki and Therapeutic Touch to lesser known techniques such as ThetaHealing, Chios, Healing Touch, Quantum Touch, Matrix Energetics, Reference Point Therapy, and DNA Activation. Some methods (like Tapas Acupressure Technique, Body Talk Therapy, and Emotional Freedom Technique) use gentle tapping of the body's energy meridians to clear blockages, while others (like percussion therapy) continually tap the muscle fascia to smooth out tissue, relieving muscle spasm. Some systems (like magnet therapy) use magnets, or implement machines that measure or move energy (like Biofeedback). Other methods that measure energy include dowsing and applied kinesiology. Some practitioners use mechanically or organically generated sound waves, like crystal or Tibetan healing bowls, or even cymatic therapy.

While a spiritual practice is not needed to practice energy medicine, some practitioners feel comfortable in a religious or spiritual framework. They may call what they do "spiritual healing," be it the laying on of hands or even simple healing prayer. Some feel more comfortable with what could be termed "shamanic journeying," including but not limited to cord cutting, imprint removal, and soul retrieval techniques. More accepted, established systems could certainly fall in this category, too, including acupuncture (or acupressure), craniosacral therapy, homeopathy, and flower essence therapy. Others may use techniques like hypnosis, dreamwork, or even Neuro-Linguistic Programming, and it certainly does not end here—it seems an energetic healing format is (re)discovered all the time! You may notice that many of these methods can be used in person or in a distance healing situation.

The term *energy* as defined here is simply vitalizing life force. It is unseen but felt, and similar in concept to what is called *qi* or *chi* in Eastern cultures and *prana* in India. Before we experience physical disease, we have the experience in our energy field first. This usually occurs through a form of trauma, remembered or not. If this is not processed on the energetic level, and the cells are not returned to their original state, then it becomes a physical condition, or dis-ease (lack of ease). If the issue is still not properly addressed, it is possible to pass this energetic imprint to our descendants, which is what we could call genetic disease.

Once the issue manifests physically, it is more difficult to return the body to its prior healed state. This is because, while the original energetic issue still needs to be addressed, there are also now physical symptoms that need to be addressed, pain being one of the largest. So basically, energy medicine addresses this traumatic imprint removal on an energy level, a step that is often forgotten in the healing process.

Herbalists already have many techniques for relieving the physical issues of disease, through the use of herbs and accompanying therapies that provide (a) detoxification and (b) nourishing substance for rebuilding, and some herbs could be used for pain management as well. However, when herbalism is combined with an energy medicine therapy that addresses the underlying issues by loosening and releasing the original trauma, this can greatly speed up the detoxification and regeneration process, which in turn lessens the time needed for the herbal therapies to work, all while simultaneously reducing pain and other cleansing reaction symptoms! How does this work?

When the original energetic issue is released, the body then operates in a less resistant way when herbal therapies are implemented. In fact, the body actually strives to match the restored energy work. If the traumatic imprint was still there, herbal therapy alone would take much longer to correct the problem due to the body's natural resistance provided by the imprint. And even with all that progress, the disease could return due to the remaining imprint! True healing only occurs when the original traumatic imprint is cleared *and* the body fully clears and repairs the condition, preventing it from recurring.

# Types of Energy Medicine

It would be impossible to list and describe all energy medicine therapies, systems, and protocols in a short article such as this. However, the following can be a starting point to begin your own research to choose the best energy medicine method(s) to study and then integrate into your herbal practice. If it seems confusing, ask Spirit or your higher self for guidance. Often the right energy medicine methods appear to you and make themselves available when you are ready to learn and use them.

## Reiki

The word Reiki is a combination of two Japanese words: *rei*, meaning universal, spiritual, or All That Is; and *ki*, meaning the cosmic breath, energy, or life force. Reiki is a gentle energetic pain-relieving, healing, and self-improvement system. This is done by the use of certain hand positions placed near the area(s) that need healing, and it can assist in dissolving and releasing traumatic imprints. By implementing certain Reiki symbols, this healing method also works at a distance.

While anyone can do Reiki by learning placement of hands, you can enhance this ability in stages through receiving what are called "attunements." A Reiki I attunement is the beginning of a deeper awareness of energetic healing. These methods can be used on people, animals, foods, water, and, interestingly, even appliances and automobiles! A Reiki II attunement involves the learning of symbols so that healing work can be done from a distance. The continuing growth of awareness also enhances the healing ability, which could be likened to comparing a dial-up Internet connection to a broadband one. Reiki III (or Reiki Master) is where the understanding of healing energies and symbols, while always growing, is considered to be at a Master level, and this person can also now attune others to Reiki.

While these attunements bump you up to the next level in healing, you could also experience cleansing reactions as you shed your old energy and integrate the new. At one time these symbols were closely guarded, but now nearly anyone has access to them to broaden their ability to heal themselves and others. However, it is highly recommended to receive lessons and attunements from a Reiki Master with a documented lineage, since the proverbial healing pipeline could then be compared to a T1 connection!

**Body Talk Therapy**
Our bodies have energy systems called meridians, which are accessed by acupuncturists and massage therapists to release stagnant energy and restore flow. Body Talk Therapy instead uses gentle tapping or other hands-on stimulation of particular points where the body's communication is disconnected due to trauma. Through certain motions the body understands, the natural communication of these cells is reconnected. Healing then happens on its own. Other systems that are similar in nature include TATLife, Emotional Freedom Technique, Chinosis, and to some degree Polarity Therapy, Matrix Energetics, and Meridian Therapy. Donna Eden also has a wonderful system of energy medicine. The variations are great, so find the system that feels right.

**Dowsing**
Sometimes described as a "spiritual telephone," dowsing can be done with a pendulum, copper rods, or even your body. Through specific questioning, as well as implementing a system

for interpreting the answer, dowsing is an amazing way to measure energy, which can help you plan the next steps in a healing process. With more advanced techniques, you can even intend changes for a more desired outcome using these same tools (like obtaining spiritual permission to remove a trauma imprint).

As an herbalist who knew dowsing beforehand, I constantly use the pendulum to choose herbs for a situation where I am not sure of underlying causes, safest and most effective dosages/timing, and even timing for overcoming the condition. Another energetic system of measurement is Applied Kinesiology, or muscle testing. For a start on understanding the energetic causes of disease, read *You Can Heal Your Life* by Louise L. Hay or *Feelings Buried Alive Never Die* by Karol K. Truman.

### Shamanic Arts

If many of these energetic healing techniques sound too New-Agey to you, consider instead shamanic journeying. Some people use a drum and others meditation, but once a practitioner is in that healing "zone," many energetic healing techniques can be used: aura clearing, chakra balancing, trauma imprint removal, cord cutting, dreamwork, soul retrieval, and even DNA activation and repatterning. Practitioners who like this method say they are being guided by Spirit so that the right healing work happens, so no two journeys are alike. May your healing work increase exponentially!

# Four Roses: Tree Medicine from the Rose Family

### By Darcey Blue French

Everyone loves roses. They are the epitome of love, romance, friendship, affection, passion, and sweetness. Their fragrance soothes and calms and brings a smile to the face of anyone who inhales their sweetness. Roses speak to the heart.

The rose family is one of the most widespread botanical families of flowering plants on the planet. It includes everything from sweet-smelling wild roses, apples, strawberries, raspberries, cherries, and almonds to meadowsweet and cinquefoil. In fact, there are around 3,000 different plants in the rose family, many of which are well-known herbal medicines. The rose family is characterized by flowers with five petals and

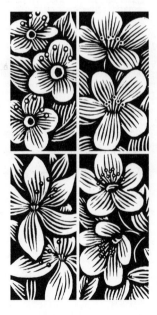

numerous stamens. Many species of rose family plants bear thorns, and may also produce edible fruits.

Rose family plants are considered astringent and are used to tone, tighten, soothe, and dry up damp, inflamed, irritated, red, or bleeding tissues. These plants are "cooling," and herbalists like to use the rose family to soothe tissues and conditions that are hot and inflamed. Rose tea may be used as a wash on sunburns or red, irritated eyes, and for cooling off on a hot summer day. Rose family plants are almost always considered nervines, calming the nervous system and the emotions.

The following rose family trees are well known for their sweet fruits, healing medicines, and beauty.

# Hawthorn

*Crataegus oxyacantha* and other spp.
**Parts used:** Berries, leaves, flowers, thorns
**Energetics:** Cooling, drying, sweet, sour, astringent
**Actions:** Stimulant, relaxant, antioxidant, tonic, nutritive, nervine, cardiac

The familiar hawthorn tree grows in hedge rows and old fields and is planted in streets and parks. It bears very sharp thorns up to one inch long! In the spring the tree is covered with white flowers that smell like rotting flesh. These stinky flowers mature into small, hard, red berries in the fall that persist on the branches long into the winter, serving as food for birds and rodents.

Hawthorn is most famous for its use as a heart tonic, addressing both the physical and emotional heart. Hawthorn is a nourishing food and medicine and is generally considered very safe. The fruits are rich in bioflavonoids, vitamins and minerals that nourish the blood and the heart by protecting from free radicals and oxidative damage. Hawthorn has been used traditionally as a tonic for weak hearts, congenital defects, and general cardiovascular health. Modern scientific study of hawthorn indicates it may be useful in moderating hypertension and cholesterol. I have often used hawthorn in formulas for such issues, but it is vitally important to realize that these conditions are complicated and must be addressed on multiple levels. There is not one herb that can cure heart disease. That said, hawthorn is a beautiful ally to protect the heart. I feel generally comfortable recommending hawthorn to people on other cardiovascular medications (excluding Coumadin or other blood thinners) as a food herb, but it is prudent and important for these folks to monitor their cardiovascular health regularly. Since hawthorn may decrease the need for medications, they should be monitored and adjusted as needed.

The fruit is commonly used, but hawthorn leaves and flowers are just as potent. They lend themselves readily to tea/infusion, whereas the fruit needs to be cooked a long time to extract the medicinal benefits. I personally like to make a combined medicine with fruit, leaf, and flower all in the same bottle. You may tincture leaf and flower in the spring, and tincture fruit in the fall, and combine the two tinctures, or tincture them dried and combine in the same jar.

It is important to remember that hawthorn is tonic and astringent and generally appropriate for folks who lack tone in the cardiovascular system. This may manifest as a weak heart, either energetically or physically. One may be pale, easily winded, or have poor circulation to the external parts of the body, because the tissues are flaccid and weak. Astringent tonics can help to tighten, tone, and strengthen such tissues to improve circulation.

Hawthorn is a remarkable ally for what the Chinese call "disturbed shen." *Shen* is the word used for spirit, the spirit that resides in the heart and makes up our mental/emotional/spiritual state of mind. We understand this in the West when we speak of heartsickness or heartbreak. What we feel with our hearts can result in a strong physical sensation in that area, such as an ache, palpitations, emptiness, or pressure. When our spirit is disturbed, the signs are anxiety, restlessness, nightmares, dreaminess/fantasy, insomnia, heartsickness or heartache, fear, panic, or trauma/PTSD. Hawthorn is a wonderful remedy in these cases. Hawthorn is useful to strengthen the physical action of the heart, and in asthmatics to improve oxygenation of the blood and breath strength. It will soothe and calm the spirit. An asthma attack may be clearly associated with disturbed shen or can result in such. It results in panic, fear, poor sleep, pressure, and often a disembodiment or tendency to get lost in "other worlds" or appear to be "taken by the Faerie."

Hawthorn is an powerful ally to anyone suffering in a situation where their heart needs extra protection emotionally and spiritually. This calming nervine brings the heart and spirit back into alignment; improves circulation of blood, oxygen, and life force; and restores balance and strength to the spirit and heart. Next time you are feeling heartache, add some hawthorn leaf and flower to your tea with something extra sweet-smelling, like linden or rose. It soothes and comforts and heals the ache. You can also sip a hawthorn berry cordial, or use small doses of the elixir or even hawthorn flower essence.

**Preparations and Dosage**

*Fresh plant:* 1 part plant by weight to 2 parts alcohol by volume, in 50% alcohol. Tincture different parts (flowers, leaves, and fruits) and mix together.

*Dry plant:* 1 part plant to 5 parts alcohol, 50% alcohol. Blend fruits, flowers, and leaves together.

Either way, fresh or dried, you may turn it into an elixir with the addition of ⅓ pint honey, using sweet brandy if desired.

*Dose:* 2–30 drops, 3 times a day. Many herbalists have noted that small doses (8–10 drops) are just as or even more effective than large doses of hawthorn.

*Infusion/decoction:* 1 tablespoon per pint of water. Steep or simmer low for 30 minutes. Take up to 16 ounces per day.

# Wild Cherry, Black Cherry, Choke Cherry

*Prunus serotina* and *Prunus virginiana*
**Parts used:** Bark, twig, flower
**Energetics:** Cool, dry, bitter, aromatic, astringent
**Actions:** Astringent, antitussive, stimulant, relaxant, tonic, heat-clearing

Wild cherry trees can easily be identified by the long, dangling racemes of sweet almond cherry-scented blossoms in early summer, followed by clusters of ruby red fruits about ½ inch in diameter with a large, hard seed. The bark of young cherry trees is smooth, shiny, and maroon or brown with prominent lenticels.

Wild cherry bark is best known as a remedy for spasmodic, irritated, hacking coughs. Just like the red cherry fruits, people who need cherry bark for their cough often have cherry-red cheeks or face from the incessant hacking and constant effort, and often have trouble sleeping as the cough worsens when they lie down. Cherry bark is best used for nocturnal cough, to aid rest, and to sedate coughs that are unproductive and tiring. Productive coughs, characterized by the healthy expelling of mucus, do not need the sedative properties of cherry. Cherry bark for coughs can be used as a tincture, a tea made in cold water, or syrup.

Cherry bark is a gentle stimulant and tonic for the digestive system and can be helpful for upset stomachs with sourness, heat, and diarrhea. Cherry is best when there is no dry condition such as constipation in the digestive system, because it tends to be astringent and drying. It is a gentle and aromatic bitter as well, and stimulates overall digestive secretions and function.

Cherry bark and flowers are sedative to the nervous and cardiovascular systems. In fact, cherry can put some people right to sleep. This is very helpful with all-night coughing to calm the cough and promote sleep. But use caution recommending cherry if the person needs to drive, operate machinery, or otherwise be alert. Cherry slows and steadies the heart rate and circulation. This is helpful for cases of anxiety and nervousness with a racing heart, tightness in the chest, and a reddish color in the face. Tincture will act quickly and is preferable to waiting for a cup of tea when you are already anxious.

I have found the cherry blossom and twig elixir harvested in spring to be remarkably effective as a sedative for that spasmodic, irritated cough, and even better than the bark for addressing heart excitability and anxiety or emotional excitability and irritability.

**Preparations and Dosage**

*Fresh flower and twig elixir:* 1 part flower/twig by weight to 2 parts alcohol by volume, in 40% brandy, and add ⅓ part by volume of honey. *Dose:* 20–30 drops up to 6 times a day. Or 5 drops every 15–30 minutes as needed for cough, racing heart, anxiety.

*Dry twig/bark tincture:* 1 part twig/bark by weight to 5 parts alcohol by volume, in 50% vodka. *Dose:* 15–30 drops, 4 times a day. Or 5 drops every 15–30 minutes.

*Cold infusion:* 1 ounce crushed bark/twig in 1 pint cold water. Macerate 4 hours. Give 4-ounce doses. Up to 16 ounces daily.

# Peach

*Prunus persica*
**Parts used:** Leaf, twig, flower
**Energetics:** Cool, moist, aromatic, bitter, sweet
**Actions:** Relaxant, tonic, sedative, heat clearing, carminative, demulcent

The peach tree has a long history of cultivation by humans and is almost always found as a tree planted in orchards and gardens, though I have found peach trees growing in campgrounds or picnic areas in unlikely settings, likely from pits discarded years ago by human visitors. The entire tree smells strongly of sweet peach and almond. The tree is covered in luscious, fragrant pink blossoms in the spring, followed by shiny, elongated oval leaves, and in late summer the prized fuzzy orange and ruby sweet peaches.

Peach, besides being a decidedly decadent and delicious cooling summer fruit, is a supreme remedy for hot, dry, irritated, and inflamed tissues, especially mucous membranes (digestive tract, urinary tract, respiratory tract). This herb is not generally available in herbal commerce, so you will want to find an organic peach tree near you.

Peach leaf can be applied to almost any situation with heat and dryness. Heat in the digestive tract can show up as redness on the tip of the tongue, heartburn, redness in the face, and nausea. Peach is excellent at quelling nausea that doesn't respond to other herbs. (If ginger doesn't work, try peach.) Peach leaf tincture is often helpful in morning sickness when taken in small, frequent doses, especially when ginger isn't helping or well tolerated. It is a lovely remedy to calm inflamed and irritated gastric tissues resulting from food allergies, irritable bowel syndrome, colitis, and so on. Peach leaf is a good tonic beverage tea for generally hot constitutions in summertime to keep cool. I often blend a little peach leaf with green tea for this.

Peach leaf tea can be helpful for chronic heartburn/gastroesophageal reflux disease, when used on a daily basis over time. It sometimes helps to relieve acute heartburn, though I find apple leaf tea more effective. Peach leaf can be combined with meadowsweet, peppermint, chamomile, marshmallow, and walnut leaf to soothe heartburn and irritated, inflamed digestive tissues.

Peach leaf is a remarkably good remedy for insect bites and stings. It relieves the itch and stinging of a simple mosquito or ant bite all the way up to scorpion stings and spider bites. I've used fresh chewed peach leaves as a poultice, or peach leaf tincture mixed with clay and placed on the bite.

I like to harvest peach leaves anytime in summer, taking small leaf clusters from lateral twigs. These are best tinctured fresh or dried completely and very carefully. Placing them flat in a single layer in a basket or box top works. If you harvest flowers and twigs, again, only harvest from lateral branches and clip cleanly to avoid damaging the remaining branch. I harvest twigs the size of my pinky finger or less. These are best tinctured fresh, as the blossoms don't last long dried, and fall apart easily.

Because peach leaf medicine is not commercially available, the best way to get it is to harvest it yourself. I've found organic orchards are often happy to let me pick leaves from their trees if I am careful. Peach trees can be grown at home, too, so you may want to plant one yourself!

## Preparations and Dosage

*Infusion:* The best infusion of peach leaf is a cold water infusion. Crush ½ ounce or a good-sized handful of dried peach leaves in a pint jar. Pour cool water over and steep for 4 hours (no longer, and keep cool, not in the sun!). Give 4 ounces, 3–5 times a day.

I have used small amounts of peach leaf in hot infusion: 1 tablespoon or less of peach leaf in a pint of hot water with green tea, lemongrass, rose, cherry, etc. These I steep for only 10 minutes, and drink fresh. The flavor of the cold infusion is much better, as the hot water pulls out more bitter compounds, but the hot version can be a nice drink to enjoy from time to time.

*Tincture or elixir:* Fresh leaf, twig, and flower tincture is quite a divine little medicine, sweet, aromatic, and bitter. It can quell nausea quite quickly in 5–10 drop doses. This small dose is safe for early pregnancy nausea. Do not give large doses of this in pregnancy. If it doesn't help in the small dose, more won't make it work any better. This is great to try with belly upsets for kids as well, but again, they don't need large doses.

*Fresh plant tincture:* 1 part plant by weight to 2 parts alcohol by volume, in 40% or 50% brandy or vodka, and add ⅓ part by volume of honey if you want to make a sweet elixir.

# Apple

*Malus spp.*
**Parts used:** Leaves, bark, fruit
**Energetics:** Cool, dry, bitter, astringent (fruit), sweet, sour
**Actions:** Tonic, febrifuge, astringent, lymphatic, nutritive

Apples have a history and biology deeply connected with humans over millennia. Wild apples were certainly used as sources of food and medicine in pre-agricultural times, but it was with the advent of agriculture and the knowledge of plant breeding that apples as we know them came into existence.

*Malus sylvestris* is the wild apple of Europe, bred into numerous domesticated and hybridized varieties (*Malus domestica*). The leaves are oval with rounded teeth, and are distinctly woolly and light on the bottom, and dark green and smooth on the top. Apples have white or pink flowers in the spring, followed by numerous green, red, or yellow fruits which can be small or large, sour or sweet. They grow wild on roadsides, in irrigation ditches, and on edges of fields.

Everyone knows the phrase "An apple a day keeps the doctor away." I'm not sure I'd go so far as to say apple is a panacea, but it is certainly well worth considering as useful medicine and nourishing food, and is underutilized by modern herbal enthusiasts.

Everyone is familiar with the sweet apple fruit, and most also know the sour crab apple. For medicinal purposes, we can use the fruit of either tree. Apples are very nourishing and are rich in minerals and vitamins: magnesium, calcium, potassium, phosphorus, vitamin C, and folate. Apple fruits are sweet, sour, astringent, and cooling. Raw apple is considered a mild laxative and is useful to address chronic constipation, due to the benefits of fiber, pectin, and minerals. Likewise, fiber and pectin are useful in addressing limited bouts of diarrhea or loose stools, as the astringency is beneficial in toning up the bowels. Applesauce has been used to alleviate diarrhea with the BRAT diet: bananas, rice, applesauce, and toast.

For some folks, raw apples can be hard to digest, and cooked apples are often a better way to eat them. They can be roasted, baked, or stewed. Crab apples should generally be cooked before using in food or medicine. My favorite recipe for baked apples is with cinnamon, ghee or butter, walnuts, and raisins or dried cranberries. I core the apples, leave them whole otherwise, fill the centers with a mix of the above, cover with foil or a lid, and bake on low to medium for an hour and a half or two hours, until the apples are soft, the skins have cracked, and the apple juice fills the pan and is bubbling. Yum! Talk about healing food!

Baked apples are generally well tolerated and easily digested and can be used as a convalescence food. Apple water (water remaining from stewing apples) is also given during fever; it is nourishing, with plenty of minerals, sweet, tasty, and comforting, and not too heavy. It is especially nice as a cooling remedy when the tongue and face are red and hot or as a cooling beverage in summer. Diluted apple cider may be used as well.

Apple leaf and bark are also useful medicines, but are directly therapeutic as opposed to nourishing. There is little in the way of recorded use of leaf and bark, but I will share here what I have learned and tried myself.

In his most famous work, *The English Physician*, Nicholas Culpeper writes of using the leaves boiled for heat in the stomach and liver that cause outbreaks on the lips: "The Leavs boyled and given to drink in hot Agues, where the heat of the Liver and Stomach causeth the Lips to break out, and the Throat to grow dry, harsh and furred, is very good to wash and gargle it withal, and to drink down som." By this I take it he means herpes cold sores, or any other hot condition in the liver and stomach. Boiled apple leaf tea is cooling and astringent and wonderful to soothe a sore, hot throat as a gargle.

Heat in the stomach and liver can also present as heartburn, acid reflux, or general burning sensations anywhere in the digestive tract. Appalachian herbalist Tommie Bass is recorded to have used apple leaf tea or syrup or bark tea or syrup when leaves weren't available for heartburn and acid stomach. I have found apple leaf tea to be helpful for heartburn. Bitter and astringent, leaves and bark will tone up and improve digestive secretions and tissue integrity overall. They may be useful for chronic cases and limited bouts of diarrhea or loose stools as well.

In *Sauer's Herbal Cures* by William Woys Weaver, American Colonial herbalist John Sauer claimed spleen effects from the fruit: "Cider pressed from very ripe sweet apples and freshly fermented may be boiled to a syrup with loaf sugar. When several spoonfuls of this are taken at a time, the syrup is quite useful against splenetic disorders, for strengthening the heart, and for dispelling faintings or palpitations, as well as melancholies caused by grief and hard times."

All parts of the plant can make a useful wash or poultice for red, inflamed, irritated skin conditions, including burns, bites, scalds, weepy rashes, minor bleeding from cuts and scrapes, sore and red eyes, and sore throats. Its toning astringent properties plus the cooling effects are helpful for these red, hot conditions.

Apple leaves aren't often found for sale in herbal commerce, so you will need to pick your own. Pick apple leaves in early summer when fully developed. You might be able to convince your local apple grower to let you harvest from unsprayed trees. In many areas of the world, wild, uncultivated apples grow where they like. They may not fruit or have palatable fruit, but their leaves and bark are very useful medicinally.

Harvest twigs and leaves from lateral branches. Twigs can be harvested anytime, but are best after flowering. Dry flat in a well-ventilated area; do not let them ferment. Do not use when partially wilted; make sure they are fully dry. Again, use clippers to prevent damage to branches when harvesting twigs. If you harvest or prune back a larger branch, strip the bark when fresh with a sharp fixed blade knife, working away from your body. Dry in strips and chop into smaller, manageable pieces for storage.

## Preparations and Dosages

*Apple leaf tea:* Place 2 teaspoons crushed apple leaves in 8 ounces boiled water. Steep 30 minutes. If you boil the leaves (as Culpeper states), the tea will be much more astringent and bitter. Take 4 ounces of tea, 3 times per day.

*Bark:* Works best as a decoction. Use ½ ounce bark or twigs in 1 quart water, and simmer on low for 10–20 minutes. You may also like a cold infusion of the bark: powder 2 teaspoons bark, and steep in 1 pint cold water for 4 hours. Take 4 ounces, 3 times daily.

You may make a syrup with the leaf/bark tea by adding an equal portion of sugar to the resulting liquid (1 cup sugar to 1 cup tea). Add 4 ounces brandy to 1 pint syrup to preserve. Store in the fridge for up to 2–3 months.

*Dry apple bark or twig tincture:* 1 part bark/twig by weight to 5 parts alcohol by volume, in 50% vodka or brandy. Apple bark is astringent enough that you should add 10% vegetable glycerin to the volume of alcohol to prevent the tannins from precipitating out of the tincture over time. For example, use 4 ounces dried apple leaf/bark, 20 ounces brandy or vodka, and 2 ounces vegetable glycerin.

Dose for the tincture should be low: 10–20 drops, 3 times a day. I prefer tea or syrup with this plant, though, as all recorded information states to use it as a tea rather than tincture.

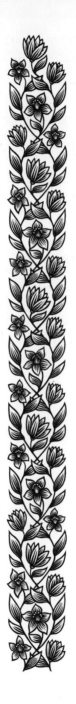

# Herb Crafts

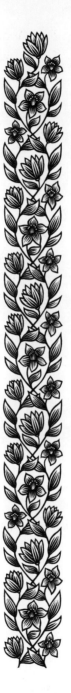

# Perfect Carrier Oils
# for Your Herbs

### ᨓ by JD Hortwort ᨓ

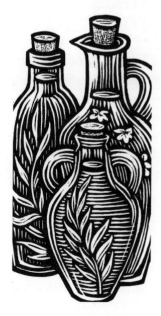

S oft, luxurious, scented oils for the
bath. Deliciously infused herbal
oils for a salad in the depth of winter.
Home-crafted herbal oil infusions
can be a blessing during times of
stress and a joy when dining—but
only if prepared properly.

Whether you want herbal oils
for the palette or for the body, using
the right oil for the job will ensure
better results.

## Getting Started

The methods discussed here are infusions and macerations. An infusion
is made by steeping plant material in
a solution, usually water, alcohol, or
oil. It can be a cold or hot infusion.
Every time you make a cup of tea, you

make a hot infusion. If you have ever mixed together vinaigrette, you've made a cold infusion. Infusions typically need to steep for a month or more.

A maceration is made by heating the oil and then adding the plant material. Heat serves to rupture the plant cell wall, thereby releasing the needed plant oils. This type of process requires care so the essential oils in the plant are not lost due to evaporation. Too much heat or improper handling during the process, and you'll cook away the very oils you want to capture.

You may ask, if heat destroys and I can just make a cold infusion, why would I bother with the heat at all?

It's true that when working with fresh flower petals and plant leaves, the best rule of thumb is, easy does it. But sometimes, stronger measures are needed. For example, getting the compounds you want from roots or bark can be very hard to do if you just pour oil over these materials. Heat will coax the essential oils from these tougher plant materials.

Also, some oils are solid at room temperature. Shea butter is a good example. You can do an effleurage, but this is very time consuming and labor intensive. Effleurage is a process that has been around for a long time but was perfected in France in the late 1800s. A solid fat is spread over a glass plate and held at room temperature. The plant material, usually flower petals, is embedded in the fat. The plate is held for days or weeks, depending on the material being used. After a set amount of time, the old plant material is removed and new material is added. With time, the essential plant oils fully impregnate the fat.

If you don't have the time or space to do an effleurage, it's better to go with a maceration. When deciding whether to do a maceration or an infusion, ask yourself a few questions. Will I be using delicate materials like thin leaves or fresh flower petals? Then an infusion is a good way to go. Do I have a lot of time? If the answer is yes, an infusion may be the best approach. Do I need the end product right away and/or am I dealing with thick leaves or roots? If so, you might consider using a maceration process. As your experience level increases, you'll soon learn which process works best for you.

## Notes on Preparation

First buy from reputable sources. The best oils will be cold-pressed, not rendered through solvents or by heat. Chemical solvents leave behind traces, which you may not want to ingest or absorb through the skin. The high heat used in heat-extraction methods can destroy or change the molecular structure of the oil being extracted. Either way, you lose the benefits you hoped to gain by selecting the right carrier oil for your mixture.

Good, cold-pressed oils are expensive. The temptation to adulterate or misrepresent a product is high. This is another reason to deal only with reputable suppliers. You should also look for suppliers that use sustainable methods of production.

Don't use copper, aluminum, or iron pots in your preparations. Use enamel or glass cooking implements. These are sometimes called nonreactive receptacles. Steel cookware or glazed clay containers are also appropriate because these surfaces will not interact with the herbs or oils you will be using.

Dry storage jars completely. Leftover moisture can contaminate your creation. Try placing containers in the oven at 150°F for 5 minutes prior to filling. Cool and then use.

Gift stores often sell pretty bottles stuffed with various fruits or vegetables and covered in oil. Check the label. It will frequently indicate this container is for looks only, not for consumption. The reason is that light can destroy the beneficial aspects of an infusion.

The best way to store infused oils is out of the light, not on a sunny windowsill. Pick colored glass containers with good lids to hold your creations. Placing the container in a cool place is best. Refrigerating the infusion will prolong the shelf life. If you need to warm it before use, transfer the necessary amount to a small bottle. Cap the bottle and set it in a hot water bath for 10–15 minutes. Then use as directed.

Oxygen is the enemy when it comes to infused oils. When oxygen comes in contact with plant material in oil, the plant stuff begins to mold. This can ruin a preparation. Use a large enough container to be able to top the herbs with at least an inch of carrier oil.

During the assembly stage and when bottling up the infusion or maceration, use a wooden spoon or chopstick. Stir, poke, and mix until you are certain there is no air left between the leaves and petals. Once again, if oxygen bubbles are left in among the plant material, a good chance exists that your creation will mold.

The risk of contamination goes up once you've opened the container and started using the oil. It's that pesky oxygen again. Refrigerating the bottle of oil helps. Another way to preserve your prepared oils is to store them in wine bottles. Pick the dark green or blue ones. Instead of using a cork, do what wine lovers do. Use a stopper that allows you to pump the extra air out of the bottle after each opening. Inexpensive wine stoppers and pumps are available at most department stores and wine shops.

Combining oils can extend the life of certain carriers. For example, grape seed oil is a great carrier for cosmetic products, but it has a short shelf life. You can extend the life of your creation with the inclusion of at least 10 percent olive oil or up to 10 percent wheat germ oil. You get the anti-microbial benefits of these additions without the heavy smell of either. You can also add 1–2 capsules (1000 mg) vitamin E to 1 ounce carrier oil to get a similar benefit. Ten drops of myrrh tincture per ounce will not harm your creation and will also extend the shelf life.

Also, don't forget that some people are allergic to nut oils like almond, peanut, or coconut. Don't use nut oils if there is a possibility of causing an allergic reaction in the user.

## The Right Oil

If the world was a simple place, now would be the time to tell you one or two oils work for everything you want to do, every time. Sadly, we all know the world is not a simple place.

Some oils are too heavy for certain applications. Others are too light. Some have a very short shelf life. While most oils are edible, that doesn't mean you would want to taste them in your creations. Certain oils work better in combinations than others.

We can rule out one type of oil immediately. Petroleum oils have their place, in a pinch. After a long day working in red clay in the garden, petroleum jelly can relieve dry hands by trapping moisture in the skin. But health concerns tend to rule them out for long-term use. Oils derived from petroleum products are drying to the skin. They will destroy fat-soluble vitamins such as vitamins A, D, E, F, and K as they are metabolized.

Olive oil is the standard for many herbalists and kitchen connoisseurs. Extra virgin olive oil is a special favorite. Plus olive oil, because of its chemical makeup, has a very long shelf life. It can be stored without refrigeration for up to a year.

As an edible oil, olive oil is packed with vitamins, minerals, and—very important for those with heart conditions—essential fatty acids. Medicinally, olive oil is a natural go-to for relieving inflamed skin. It has anti-microbial properties. Mothers-to-be have used it for generations to help prevent stretch marks. Olive oil can be a carrier for preparations to alleviate sprains, bruises, and rheumatism.

The concern with olive oil is its classic smell and taste. The aroma of olive oil in a salad dressing is wonderful, but in a facial cream, not so much. You can still get the benefits of olive oil in your concoctions if you blend it at a rate of 10 percent olive oil to 90 percent secondary oil.

Grape seed oil is a lighter oil that will let the flavors of herbs come through in a marinade or salad dressing. Because it is so light, grape seed oil easily penetrates the skin, making it great for cosmetic purposes. In particular, grape seed oil is mildly astringent. Use it in preparations for acne. The biggest drawback of grape seed oil is its short shelf life. Combining it with olive oil will help combat this shortcoming. If using it alone or with other short-life oils, mix small batches that will be utilized quickly.

Almond oil is a classic oil for cosmetics because it is easily absorbed into the skin. Many associate the fragrance of almond oil with their grandmothers' lotions. Its penetrating aspects make it a favorite among massage therapists. Its omega-6 and omega-9 content gives this oil an immune-boosting benefit. Use almond oil as a carrier in preparations for dry scalp, dry hair, and eczema. A word of caution here: Sweet almond oil is edible; bitter almond oil is not. Also, the fragrance of almond oil is a selling point, but only if you want that sweet aroma coming through in the final preparation.

Sesame seed oil will hold up in preparations without lending a conflicting fragrance. It is edible, readily available, and inexpensive to use. Sesame seed oil works well as a skin moisturizer. It is a natural in preparations for rheumatic conditions, eczema, psoriasis, and just general dry skin due to the high content of lecithin, Vitamin B complex, Vitamin E, calcium, magnesium, and phosphorus. As a massage oil, sesame seed oil is thought to relieve stress and anxiety and is safe enough for use on infants. While sesame seeds go rancid quickly at room temperature (roughly six months), sesame seed oil has a shelf life comparable to olive oil.

Jojoba oil is a popular carrier for skin and hair applications. Technically it is not an oil; it is a wax. It is relatively stable in storage, although it won't hold as long as olive oil at room temperature. Use it in preparations to restore moisture to the skin and balance natural body oil production. Its use for control of acne is well known, but keep in mind, a little goes a long way. Over-apply and you may end up complicating an acne problem. Jojoba can also be used in natural shaving cream mixtures.

When you want to turn your herbal oil into an ointment, try mixing it with shea butter. Experts will tell you shea butter is not an oil; it is a fat. We're parsing words here, but oil is liquid at room temperature, while a fat is solid. If the room temperature is up to around 98 degrees, shea butter will become liquid. This is good. It means shea butter melts at average body temperatures, making it a very good carrier for body creams.

The proportion of shea butter to carrier oil will vary depending on how solid you want the end product to be. A general rule of thumb would be 1 part carrier oil to 5 parts shea butter. Of course, you can also make a maceration with just shea butter. Gently heat the butter to a liquid state, then incorporate herbs and allow them to steep. Leaves and flower petals can be gently steeped for 2–4 hours. Roots and barks may require overnight holding in a crockpot.

Remove the plant material. Repeat the process if you want a more intense blend. At the final stage, remove the plant material and allow the shea butter to solidify. If you want a lighter texture, put the herbal concoction in a glass bowl. Nest this in a large bowl of ice. Use a mixer to whip the butter to a lighter consistency as it resolidifies.

These are some basic, readily available carrier oils. With Internet trade and all of the global markets open to us, many more beneficial oils are coming on the market. Do your research and feel free to experiment. The end result is sure to be tasty to eat or delightful to use.

# Herbal Baths

### ⁓ by Laurel Reufner ⁓

Few things are as enjoyable as soaking in a nice, warm tub. Except perhaps a soak in a nice, warm tub that's had some lovely, scented goodness added to it. An herbal bath can be many things: relaxing, soothing, healing, even magical. (Scott Cunningham's books *The Magical Household* and *The Complete Book of Incense, Oils & Brews* contain some excellent information on magic and the bath.)

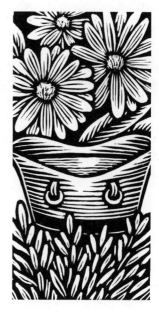

There are a couple different ways to prepare an herbal bath. The fastest and easiest—my favorite—is simply to place your ingredients in a cloth or small bag and toss it in the water. Allow the herbs to steep both while the water is running and during your soak and you're good to go. Some herbal baths, however, do better if you steep them on the stove as a heated infusion before adding the final brew to the water. Sometimes you need everything already steeped and ready to work before you get into the water. My sunburn bath is one of those formulas.

## Herbal Bath Ingredients

Let's start with a list of some useful bath additives, beginning with the herbs. I like to have these on hand for a variety of uses in both the kitchen and the bath.

### Calendula

Calendula possesses anti-inflammatory and antiseptic properties, making it good for healing. Actually, the herb is good for all types of skin complaints, including acne, eczema, and most skin rashes as well. It also works as a bit of an astringent. I've used balms containing calendula on all types of skin conditions with good results, including, in a pinch, a really nasty sunburn. It's a great herb to have on hand.

### Chamomile

Like many of the herbs on this list, chamomile is a soothing, relaxing herb that can help make your skin glow. The herb is also cleansing and can cause a purifying sweat when taken internally. In the bath, it can be useful for sunburn or stiff, sore muscles.

### Eucalyptus

A soak with this herb can relieve aching joints. It also has antiseptic, antiviral, and deodorizing properties. Eucalyptus is known mainly for its expectorant properties, which also holds true when used in the bath.

## Ginger

Ginger possesses stimulating properties that can be quite useful in some healing baths, especially when dealing with sore muscles or colds and congestion. It also has a lovely smell.

## Lavender

One of the top herbs everyone should have on hand, lavender has several useful properties that can be used in an herbal bath. It has a tonic effect on the nervous system, helping balance a person's nerves and emotions—soothing, calming, and relaxing them. Lavender is also incredibly antiseptic, antiviral, and antibacterial.

## Lemon Balm

Lemon balm can help open the pores and promote perspiration, making it good at cleansing the skin of toxins. Personally I've never used that strong of a concentration in my bath, so I tend to find it calming and soothing, with a pleasant lemon scent that can help you get your oomph back after a long day. This herb is also good for soothing unpleasant bug bites.

## Oats

Oats are very soothing to dry skin as well as skin conditions such as eczema. For bath purposes, you will want to make an infusion on the stove and then strain and add the water to your bath. If not using a colloidal oatmeal, like Aveeno, confine it to a bath bag of some sort. Do not put non-colloidal oats loose into your bath water, or you'll have one heck of a mess to clean up and you may ruin your plumbing. Oats are a nice additive to the tub for itchy skin.

## Peppermint

This aromatic herb has wonderful soothing and cooling properties in the bath. Those same aromatic properties also make it great for baths when you're suffering from a cold or headache. Peppermint is also nice to use for general aches and pains as well as itchy, dry skin.

## Rosebuds/Petals

Rose petals are my other favorite herb to have on hand and are just plain lovely in the bath to help cheer the spirit and relax the body. They're very comforting for a soak. Rose petals also work as an astringent and are very cleansing to the skin, helping soothe rashes and inflammations and helping give your skin a glow.

## Rosemary

Rosemary works as an astringent in the bath, helping soothe skin breakouts due to eczema and acne.

## Thyme

Thyme is very refreshing in your bath water. It's also useful as an antifungal and can help soothe insect bites.

## Baking Soda

Baking soda is another nice addition for softening your skin. It's also a nice addition to help ease the tired body after a busy day. Baking soda is not quite as drying as Epsom salt.

## Epsom Salt

Epsom salt helps soothe tired muscles. It is also good for your health, since there are studies that show many Americans are deficient in magnesium. One of the best ways to increase your magnesium intake is actually by adding a cup of Epsom salt to the bath and enjoying a good soak. The magnesium is better absorbed this way than by an oral supplement.

### Powdered Milk

Powdered milk is a lovely addition to the bath, helping to soften and moisturize the skin. It's a very soothing addition to any bath, helping leave your skin silky smooth.

### Sea Salt

Salt has a softening effect on water. Left undissolved, it makes for a great scrub and exfoliant as well. The only catch is that salt can be very drying to the skin. Table salt will work as well as sea salt in a pinch.

## Other Useful Items

Here are some other useful items to have on hand when mixing up your herbal concoctions.

### Muslin Bags

Simple muslin bags are very easy to whip up with a sewing machine, although you might be able to find some already made at your local health food store, especially if they deal in bulk herbs. Another good option for making bath bags is heat-sealed tea bags, the kind where you fill the bags with your own choice of teas and then iron them shut.

### Washcloths

Using squares of washcloths is probably the easiest way to make a quick bath bag. Simply place your materials in the middle of the cloth, pull up the edges, and fasten shut with some string or a rubber band and you're good to go.

### Small Coffee Grinder

A small coffee grinder is the best way I've found to reduce your herbal ingredients to fine bits. Nothing fancy is required; just a small, simple, countertop grinder will work. A grinder can often be bought for around twenty dollars. If you don't mind having to put in the added effort and time, a mortar and pestle will work as well. The mortar and pestle might be the better option if you want to add some magical energies to the water along with the beauty and health properties of your ingredients. You can add in the energies as you grind the herbs.

### Measuring Spoons

Measuring spoons will help you get the proportions of your bath mixture just right.

### Small Glass Bowl

You'll need something in which to mix all your ingredients, and a glass bowl is ideal. I'm not a big fan of metal or plastic, although they'll work in a pinch.

### Glass or Ceramic Cooking Pot

Some herbal baths work better if you infuse a pot of water on the stovetop and then add it to your bath. With a glass or ceramic pan, you don't have to worry about anything leeching out of the metal and into your bath water.

### Storage Containers

Several bath bags can be made up at once, making it easier to simply grab one and toss it into the tub when you desire. Storing them in a simple plastic bag or resealable container will do the trick. If you're giving some bath bags as a gift, an inexpensive jar can be easily decorated and will look quite pretty.

# The Recipes

Here are a few recipes to get you started. A good rule of thumb when mixing up the formulas is to allow for between ¼ and ½ cup mixture total, unless otherwise noted in the recipe. I hope you enjoy these.

### Sunburn Bath

Several years ago, my husband got the worst sunburn. A good chunk of his body was beet red. Turning to my herbals, this is the formula I came up with, and my husband can attest to its wonderful effectiveness. Yes, regular tea bags or vinegar in the bath will also soothe a sunburn, but I'm not sure they'll do the trick on a really bad sunburn quite as well as this recipe will.

    1 part chamomile

    1 part crushed juniper berries

    1 part lavender buds

    1 part rose petals

    1 part witch hazel

Add the ingredients—about ⅛ cup each—to 2 cups water and prepare as an infusion. Allow to soak for 15–20 minutes. Pour the liquid into a cool bath and add ½ cup finely ground oatmeal. Soak in the water for about half an hour and finish by gently drying off and applying a good lotion.

### Orange Spice

    1 loosely filled cup orange peel

    1 stick cinnamon

    ⅛ cup fresh ginger, cut up into small pieces

    2 cups water

Bring the ingredients to a boil on the stove, then turn it off and let the mixture steep for 20 minutes. Strain and add to your bath along with a packet of dried milk. The mix of scents will help revive your energy and clear your head.

### Lavender Dreams

- 1 part lavender
- 1 part rose petals
- ½–1 cup baking soda

Mix the ingredients together in a small bowl, add to a muslin bag or washcloth, then toss it into your bath water. Enjoy.

### Cold Comfort

- 2 tablespoons eucalyptus
- 4 tablespoons rosemary
- 4 tablespoons lavender buds
- 2 tablespoons rosebuds
- 2 cups water

Bring the water to a boil and turn off the heat. Put the herbs in a muslin bag, then add to the water and allow to steep for 20 minutes. Add to a nice, warm bath and soak. Try to breathe in the fumes from the herbs to help with the healing.

### Soothe Your Itchies

- 1 tablespoon calendula
- 1 tablespoon rosebuds/petals
- 2 tablespoons lemon balm
- 2 tablespoons thyme

½ cup oats, or 1 packet oatmeal bath additive

½ cup powdered milk

Combine everything except the milk and oatmeal (if using the colloidal oats) in a muslin bag and add to warm bath water. Allow to steep for several minutes, then climb in and soak.

### Magnesium

1 cup Epsom salt

¼ cup of your favorite-scented herb

1 packet powdered milk

Either grind the herb to a fine powder or place in a cloth bag. Add to the bathtub, along with the milk and Epsom salt. Draw a nice, warm bath and allow yourself to soak for at least 20 minutes to give the mineral time to be absorbed by your body.

There you have it: a beginning list of herbal bath ingredients as well as some recipes to get you started. There's just one more thing to talk about before I turn you loose in your herb stash … What do you do if you can't take a bath? Can any of these herbal bath recipes still be used? Well, maybe not all of them can be converted to a shower-only situation, but yes, you can use herbal baths without the bath. The easiest method is to add the ingredients to the center of a washcloth and tie it closed. Then simply scrub yourself down with the wet washcloth while you're in the shower. A second easy method is to somehow fasten the washcloth to the showerhead so the water runs through it, picking up the herbal goodness on its way. Finally, you can make an infusion of your herbs of choice on the stovetop and allow it to cool. Then simply pour it over yourself at some point. It may not be quite as satisfying as soaking in the tub, but it will still get the job done.

Now go. Enjoy your bath!

# The Scrapbook Candle

### ☙ by Lexa Olick ❧

A candle is such a simple object. It can be created from no more than wax and a wick, yet it symbolizes so much. The flame produces a small light, which sets the perfect tone for an intimate evening. It gives us a sense of warmth and companionship. The burning candle is also a light in the darkness and a symbol of hope. For centuries, candles were placed in windows to guide loved ones home. Therefore, candles are a way to bring families closer together.

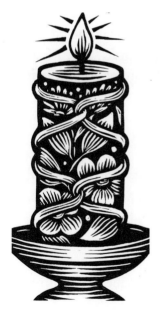

Candles hold so many memories, most notably scented candles. Their scent invokes memories of childhood, holidays, and momentous occasions. It is amazing how lighting a candle can transport us back to happier times.

We can be brought back to those same times by turning the page of a scrapbook. Scrapbooking is another way to bring people closer together. Scrapbooks document the story of a person's life. Memories are forever preserved with photos, cards, and poetry. Both scrapbooks and candles link us to our past and our happiest memories. It was only a matter of time before the two were joined together.

A scrapbook candle is a candle that tells a story. Precious memories are used to turn an ordinary candle into an object of value. It is the perfect candle to burn after you've ended a chapter in your life, such as a graduation, or to use as a centerpiece to display your life as a precious object. Flowers and herbs make the best embellishments for your candle. So many great occasions are marked by plants, such as bouquets from a wedding, herbs from a garden, or a fallen autumn leaf.

I pressed flowers before I even knew what I was doing. It started at age five. I spent my summer days scavenging through the grass. It would take me hours to find a four-leaf clover. Once I found my prize, I would slip it into the back of my diary. Life moved so fast that I could barely keep up with it by writing alone. When I discovered my diary years later, I was initially disappointed in how little I had written, but suddenly all those plants and flowers fell from the pages. I may not have documented my life through written words, but those pressed plants held so many memories of my childhood. I had a visual diary that expressed more than I could have possibly written.

Just as with a scented candle, the smell of dried herbs invokes memories. The scrapbook candle combines visual mementos with sentimental scents. It helps you to connect to people, places, and events by telling the story of your life. Many people light candles for relaxation and meditation. It only makes sense to combine them with the objects that make you happy.

Pressed flowers have always been a popular embellishment for candles. Mostly they are découpaged on top of the wax. However, the scrapbook candle is decorated with flowers, herbs, and other objects by entwining everything together with raffia. It not only gives the candle texture, but also lets you play around with your material and discover the best arrangement for your objects. Leaves can be slipped in and out of the raffia. Different materials can be added as you work. The candle may be tied with raffia ribbon, but you are not tied down to a specific order. You can alternate the objects as you work to create a candle that best tells your story.

Flowers and herbs are not the only objects you can use to decorate your scrapbook candle. You can also use small photographs, coins, poetry written on paper, or small flat stones. Essentially you can use anything that slips underneath the raffia. When it comes to plants, pressed flowers and herbs are best because they lie flat against the candle, but small sprigs work well, too. The material list that follows is just a guide. You can customize it with different items that truly express yourself.

*Materials*

    1 scented pillar candle

    6 yards raffia ribbon

    10 dried leaves of pressed herbs

    2 wallet-size photographs

    Scissors

Glass dish

¼ cup small pebbles

¼ cup buttons

¼ cup acorns

1. Cut 4 lengths of raffia ribbon that measure 1½ yards apiece.

2. Hold the lengths of raffia evenly together and find their center. Place the candle in front of you. Begin to wrap the candle at the top and work your way down. To do so, place the center of the raffia around the candle. Pull the raffia towards the back and loop the strands over one another to form an $X$ and then bring back to the front of the candle.

Continue to wrap the raffia around the candle until you reach the bottom. Once you hit the bottom, secure the raffia with a knot and trim the excess.

3. Insert herbs and photos underneath the raffia. Every time you slip an item underneath the raffia, think what each object symbolizes. Reflect on how the memories of your photos and herbs connect with the scent of the candle.

4. Fill a glass dish with pebbles, buttons, and acorns. Sit the candle in the dish. As the candle burns, the raffia loosens and allows the herbs to slip away from the candle. Keep your eyes on the candle while it is lit. You should never leave a lit candle unattended.

# Herb History, Myth, and Lore

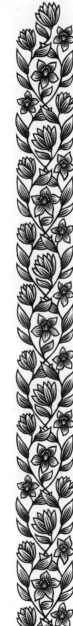

# The Golden Apples of Jotunheim

### ❧ by Linda Raedisch ❧

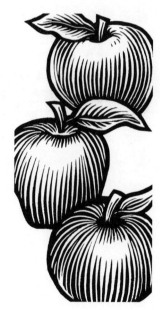

There are few landscapes as haunting as the apple orchard in winter. The bare trees against the snow resemble bronze figures of the Hindu god Shiva, twisted limbs upraised in the celestial dance. Neglect only heightens the atmosphere of mystery, for a less than well tended apple tree might offer itself as a host to parasites. Here and there we spot the unearthly glow of tiny moons against the bark's lichened patina. These are the white berries of the mistletoe. We've all heard how the Druids revered the clusters of mistletoe they found growing in oak trees, but the apple tree is actually a far more common host.

The mistletoe, with its roots in the sky, plays a prominent role in one of the most celebrated Norse myths, the Death of Balder. But we have come to hear the story of another of the Aesir, the gods who dwelt in Asgard. She is the goddess Idunn. Her name, most scholars agree, has to do with youth and rejuvenation, for her task is to keep the gods young. There she is, standing barefoot in the snow, her form half hidden by the snaking limbs of the oldest tree in the orchard. Her face is turned from us, but we can see her golden hair rippling to her ankles, her bright garment thrown carelessly over her shoulder.

One cannot imagine what one has not already seen, which is why I envision Idunn much as the artists of the nineteenth century did: young and guilelessly beautiful, dressed in what looks more like a Greek chiton or Indian sari than anything a Norse housewife might have worn. Danish artist Lorenz Froelich offers us a rather thick-limbed Idunn in green draperies, one arm threaded casually through the handle of a golden lunch pail. Idunn never goes anywhere without her apples, though sometimes she carries them in a basket and at other times a bowl. In *Prose Edda*, twelfth-century Icelandic poet Snorri Sturluson tells us that Idunn keeps her apples in a bag. Later, however, he refers to a casket made of ashwood in which the all-important apples reside.

Here within the walls of Asgard, it seems to be a box that our Idunn is carrying inside the embroidered folds of her garment. As we advance, the goddess retreats, the apples rattling noisily as her footfalls quicken over the crust of the snow. We really can't blame her for being wary, not after that episode with the jotun Thiazi. *Jotun* is almost always translated as "giant," but this is a little misleading. It is not the size of the jotnar but their wild nature that is important. The jotun creed is the antithesis of the order and discipline that (usually) reigns at Asgard. While the jotnar are dangerous, uncivilized creatures, the stories suggest that they can also be fair to look upon, and there are more than a few instances of mutual attraction between the jotnar and the gods.

Well, after a disagreement concerning some ox meat, the jotun Thiazi compelled the god Loki to deliver him the goddess Idunn along with her magical apples. The unscrupulous Loki lured Idunn outside the walls of Asgard with the promise of even better apples to be found in the forest. She should, he told her, bring her own apples along for comparison. As soon as Idunn arrived in the wood, Thiazi swooped down in the shape of an eagle, seized her, and bore her away to the wild wastes of Jotunheim. Loki eventually made good, flying to Thiazi's mountain aerie to rescue Idunn. Just in time, too, for, deprived of the apples, the gods were quickly growing old and gray. Loki returned with Idunn (apples intact), Thiazi was killed, the gods were saved, and a revenge plot on the part of Thiazi's daughter Skadi was quashed by a gesture of goodwill.

Skadi is actually my favorite character in the whole escapade. When her father was killed, she clapped on her skis, threw her braids over her shoulders, and hightailed it to Asgard to avenge him. But when she arrived, she was offered the god with the prettiest feet for a husband. Who could say no to that? Judging the Aesir by their feet and calves alone, Skadi believed she was choosing Balder (later to be slain by the mistletoe, thanks to Loki's conniving), but the winner of this unusual beauty contest turned out to be the fertility god Njord. God and jotun took a stab at married life, but Skadi was unhappy in her husband's boathouse by the sea, just as Njord was not quite comfortable in wolf-ridden Jotunheim. They parted ways, Skadi, in her snowshoes, trudging back to her ancestral home in the mountains.

You might wonder why I am running on about Skadi when it is Idunn we are pursuing across the frozen orchard. The truth is that Idunn is little more than a poster girl for everlasting youth. She has almost no backstory, and little to say or do once she has been safely returned to Asgard. If we want a really good story, we must turn to the apples themselves.

If we are to trust those nineteenth-century artists, then the apples that Idunn guards so closely are some smallish but sweet heirloom variety, such as a Spitzenberg or Danish Gravenstein. Unfortunately, those varieties date back only to the seventeenth and eighteenth centuries. Besides, if you listen closely, you will notice that the apples rolling around inside Idunn's box sound more like wooden balls than anything you might want to eat. So just what kind of apples did the skalds have in mind when they first sang of Idunn over the crackling of pips in the fire?

In Central Europe, we can trace the genetically engineered apple, or cultivar, deep into prehistory. Oetzi, the five-thousand-year-old ice mummy, had no apples in his kit or in his gut, though scientists did find the remains of wild berries and blackthorn fruits. Still, that does not mean Oetzi never tasted an apple. The Copper Age Lake Dwellers of Switzerland and southern Germany ate apples raw, roasted them, and brewed a drink from the pulp. The sites of Robenhausen and Wangen-Hinterhorn have yielded the remains of both domesticated and wild apples. We do not know if the former were bred from the latter or acquired through trade with the Mediterranean.

We do know that the apples of the Hesperides, the apples celebrated through the Roman goddess Pomona, as well as all of the varieties eaten today were bred from a wild apple of Central Asia. The Germanic tribesmen living within the bounds of the empire were quick to adopt the Romans' *Malus domestica* and incorporate it into their native religion. On the eastern shores of the North Sea we discover the goddess Nehalennia sitting beside a basket of fat, juicy apples. Though Nehalennia was a Germanic goddess, she came to enjoy the trappings of Classical civilization, including Latin inscriptions on her shrines and orchard-grown apples.

Such luxuries, however, were not yet available to the inhabitants of Barbaricum or even to the much later Vikings. The richly furnished Oseberg ship burial of 834 CE contained a fancy bucket filled with apples. The bucket, with its bands of delicate, open bronzework, is believed to be of Irish or British workmanship. One might expect to find Romano-British apples inside, but the bucket held wild apples such as one could gather easily in southern Norway.

Traveling on, we arrive outside the Danish trading hub of Haithabu. It is late summer. Wattle fences protect the kitchen gardens from the shaggy cattle now lounging in the black mud of the water meadow. Close beside the framework houses we find beds of horse beans, leeks, and a variety of herbs. Here and there is a plum tree and over there, beside that large house with all the thralls going in and out of it, is a peach tree. There are, however, no orchards, and no apple trees. But here come the children, clattering across the wooden planks laid over the mud. They have just returned from the untamed spaces beyond the earthworks, and their baskets are brimming with blackthorn fruits, elderberries, wild cherries, and, yes, wild apples. Here in the North, even the southernmost portions of the North, the diet is hardly more varied than Oetzi's was four thousand years before.

The very word, *apple*, informs us that the sacred apple of Germanic myth was not the Asian-derived *Malus domestica*. If it were, we would now expect to call our own apples by some name derived from the Latin *pomus* or the Greek *milo*. Instead, it's an apple, a word closely related to the German *apfel* and the Old Norse *epli*. This is because *apple* belongs to an especially ancient strain of Indo-European spoken north of the Alps and dubbed "Old European" by German linguist Hans Krahe. *Epli*, then, refers to *Malus sylvestris*, the wild European crabapple. But discovering that those are actually crabapples rattling around inside Idunn's gold-hinged box does not explain why the ancient Scandinavians should have chosen to celebrate such an unpalatable fruit. Could the *epli* really have been as bad as the sour marbles we now associate with the name crabapple?

Probably not. The town of Haithabu was staked out by Danish Vikings only around the year 800 CE, to be snuffed out by the Slavic Wends about two hundred years later: not quite time enough to establish the widespread Germanic tradition of the *apaldr*. *Apaldr* can mean "tree," or, specifically, "apple tree." Even more specifically, it can refer to an apple tree that stood close to the family home and was identified with both the ancestors and the family's fortunes. Archaeological evidence shows that *Malus sylvestris* enjoyed a special status not extended to other wild fruit trees. The roots were spread with dung, the branches pruned, and, if the wassailing of later centuries is any indication, the tree was sung to and offered libations. By the time the Roman apple cultivars arrived on the northern scene, shortly preceded by the plum and the peach, these hallowed native crabs had reached a semi-domesticated condition: edible, palatable (especially when fermented), but probably not delicious.

The Romans were suitably unimpressed with these Germanic apples, planting their own cultivars in neat rows throughout the empire. Unable to compete with the larger, juicier *Malus domestica*, the fruit of the ancestral tree slipped back into the forest, its seedlings quickly discarding their grudging sweetness in favor of hardiness and, true to its Rose family nature, thorns. There are now endless varieties of crabapple in the wild, but Idunn's apples are no longer to be found.

The seventeenth century presents a situation analogous to that of the Roman frontier. When the French arrived in eastern Canada, they found the Iroquois growing apples of their own, possibly a variety of *Malus coronaria*, one of the New World crabapples. Rather than just planting one or two trees outside the longhouse, the Iroquois tended whole orchards of these trees. The French acknowledged that the fruits were bigger and sweeter than the Old World crabapple. Even so, like the Romans, they set about establishing their own Rainettes and Calvilles. It was not easily done. In 1670 an Ursuline nun of Quebec wrote of how the apple trees in her convent's garden had all succumbed to the late spring ice while the native apples were unaffected.

The nuns had then to wait for new stock to arrive from France, for the only way to propagate a specific variety of apple is to take a shoot, or scion, from the desired tree and bind it to the stump, or rootstock, of another tree. The rootstock might be of another variety or even another species, such as the crabapple. Compared to the taking and planting of a seed, this seems a rather brutal method of reproduction.

The term *scion* has also come to refer to a human heir. In the Norse epic *Volsunga Saga*, the distinction between the two types of scion is often blurred. The crabapple, it must be noted, is sacred to the Anglo-Saxon god Wodan. In *Volsunga Saga*, when the grandson of Wodan's Norse counterpart, Odin, proves sterile, the god summons his wish maiden, Hljod, to help. The saga does not make it clear what a wish maiden is, but it does tell us that Hljod is the daughter of the jotun Hrimnir. Much as the jotun Thiazi turned himself into an eagle to seize Idunn and her apples, Hljod transforms herself into a crow, flies over the burial mound where sits the childless King Rerir, and drops an apple in his lap. Rerir shares the apple with his queen.

The story goes on to feature the birth of the child Volsung by Caesarean section—the scion quite literally cut from the parent—and a great hall dominated by the blossoming boughs of an *apaldr* named Barnstokkr, meaning "child trunk." For a time, the viability of the Volsung line seems assured, but Odin is continually stepping in to choose a scion, oversee the pruning of extraneous sons, and to cut down that scion when he has passed his prime. Later, the forging of Sigurd the Dragonslayer's sword from the two broken pieces of his father Sigmund's blade (which Sigmund had pulled from Barnstokkr's trunk) is reminiscent of the grafting of a scion onto a root-stock. Nowhere in the saga is the apple identified outright as a sacred symbol, perhaps because its sanctity was taken for granted by the poet and his audience.

Leaving Sigurd to his tragic end, we return to the winter orchard where Idunn's footsteps have slowed, the half-tame specimens of *Malus sylvestris* rattling less noisily in their wooden box. As we catch up with the goddess, she turns. And to our astonishment, she has grown old. Her golden hair, white now, is bound on the top of her head, and her face is as wrinkled as an old Boskoop.

This is no longer Idunn, but Frau Holle, the elderly White Lady of German fairy tale who brought forth blossoms from the apple trees in spring, who rewarded diligence and punished sloth. One of the tests she set for her would-be votaries was to present them with a groaning apple tree, heavy with fruit. She rewarded those who stopped to shake the boughs and give the tree some relief, while she punished those who ignored the tree's cries. Frau Holle may be a late expression of the goddesses Freya and Frigga. Likewise, Idunn may be only an aspect of the many-named Freya, hence her lack of dimension.

Here in the winter orchard, the trees, too, have grown old. They are no longer able to lift their limbs in the cosmic dance. Given our violently shifting climate and the dwindling number of apple varieties, it is not impossible that *Malus domestica* might someday succumb to a widespread blight, as the American chestnut did in the early twentieth century. Would this mark the end of the good eating apple?

Perhaps for a time. But listen! Someone is calling our Idunn from the boundaries of the orchard, drawing her toward the tangled wood beyond. While it is always a calamity when one of the goddesses is carried off from Asgard, female jotnar like Skadi and Hljod were welcome to enter and infuse the Aesir with new blood. At first, Skadi's mistaking of the older Njord's feet for the beautiful Balder's would seem surprising. But Skadi, forced to choose blindly as Mother Nature does, instinctively picks out the older but sturdier rootstock, the one less likely to be taken out by an infestation of mistletoe. Or is it Skadi who is the rootstock and Njord the scion? Either way, the message is clear: the apple's vitality lies in the wild. If we should ever lose our Golden Delicious, our Macintosh and Rome, we will have to return to the wilderness of Jotunheim, if there is any of it left. There, we must seek out the enduring crabapple and start all over again.

# References

Almgren, Bertil, et al. *The Viking.* Twickenham, England: Senate Publishing, 1999.

Byock, Jesse L. *The Saga of the Volsungs.* New York: Penguin Books, 1990.

Davidson, Hilda Ellis. *Roles of the Northern Goddess.* New York: Routledge, 1998. Transferred to Digital Printing 2005. Printed and bound by Antony Rowe Ltd., Eastbourne.

Erichsen-Braun, Charlotte. *Medicinal and Other Uses of North American Plants: A Historical Survey with Special Reference to the Eastern Indian Tribes.* New York: Dover Publications, 1979.

Fischer-Fabian, S. *Die Ersten Deutschen: Ueber das Raetselhafte Volk der Germanen.* Bergisch Gladbach, Germany: Bastei Luebbe, 2003.

Keller, Ferdinand. *The Lake Dwellings of Switzerland and Other Parts of Europe, Volume One*. Translated and arranged by J. E. Lee. Digitized by Google. London: Spottiswoode and Co., 1878.

Lindow, John. *Norse Mythology: A Guide to the Gods, Heroes, Rituals and Beliefs*. New York: Oxford University Press, 2001.

Renfrew, Colin. *Archaeology and Language: The Puzzle of Indo-European Origins*. New York: Cambridge University Press, 1988.

Sturluson, Snorri. *The Viking Gods*. Translated by Jean I. Young, Jon Thorisson, ed. Reykjavik, Iceland: Gudrun, 1955.

# The Artemisias

## ≫ by Suzanne Ress ≪

There are known to be more than 400 different species of the genus *Artemisia*. Most of these perennial plants have a preference for dry, rather poor soil. Many people believe that the genus *Artemisia* takes its name from the ancient Greek goddess of wild animals and the moon, Artemis. Since these plants really have nothing in common with the moon, and do not usually grow in wooded areas, it is probably more likely that the genus name comes from Queen Artemisia II of Caria (Greece/Persia), a highly skilled botanist.

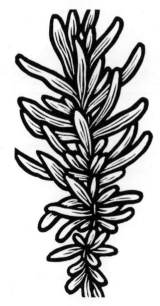

Most Artemisias have strong, often quite bitter aromas and tastes. This is due to their content of terpenoid volatile oils and sesquiterpene lactone compounds. Terpenoid oils are organic chemicals, made use of in many cases by the perfume industry, the processed food and drink industry, and by the pharmaceutical industry in antibacterial and anesthetic preparations. All aromatic herbs contain volatile essential oils, but the Artemisias have one of the highest percentages of terpenoid oils of all. Some of these are camphor, estragole, linalool, thujone, absinthol, and eucalyptol.

Sesquiterpene lactones are the organic chemical compounds that may cause allergic reactions, and are partially responsible for a plant's bitter taste. Certain sesquiterpene lactones found in members of the genus *Artemisia* have valuable antibacterial, antifungal, antiparasitic, and antihelminthic properties that modern medical science has only recently begun to discover and make use of.

The Artemisias usually flower at the end of the summer, and northern species may not flower at all. Their flowers are typically small, insignificant yellow or brownish yellow panicles (balls) at the stem tops, which cannot be pollinated by bees or other insects, but rely on wind pollination. Some Artemisias produce no seeds, and many are best propagated by division or cuttings.

The five most common species of *Artemisia* are tarragon, southernwood, mugwort, wormwood, and sagebrush.

## Tarragon

Of all the Artemisias, only tarragon is used regularly in cooking. But beware! There are two types of tarragon: French (*Artemisia drancunculus*) and Russian (*Artemisia dracunculoides*). French tarragon is, by far, superior for culinary use. If you buy a packet of tarragon seeds to plant, it won't be French tarragon, for this plant produces no seeds! If you want real French tarragon in your herb garden, you will have to buy or otherwise procure a small plant or cuttings. Even then, check a leaf or two carefully for taste and aroma.

Other common names for French tarragon are estragon, little dragon, or dragoncello. Its slender, pointy leaves have the look of a dragon's hackles, and, if you dig up the plant, its roots are twisted and curved like a dragon's tail. The flavor of French tarragon could also make one think of a cute little dragon, for it has a warm, almost liquorice-like bite to it.

The main terpenoid oil in French tarragon is estragole. This oil also occurs, in much lesser amounts, in basil, pine oil, turpentine, fennel, and anise. It is highly prized by perfumers, processed food manufacturers, and cooks everywhere. Tarragon is one of French cuisine's four *fines herbes*, which also include parsley, chervil, and chives.

French tarragon's leaves can be chopped and used fresh (but sparingly!) in fish, egg, chicken, or potato salads. A classic use for tarragon in the kitchen is in infused vinegar; add a long sprig and a peeled clove of garlic to a bottle of high-quality white wine vinegar, and leave for a month or more before using. This, combined with olive oil, is excellent on green salads or cooked vegetables such as potatoes, carrots, peas, or asparagus. Tarragon's flavor pairs very well with almost all fish or chicken dishes, but can also be tried successfully with pork, and even beef, as in béarnaise sauce. Fine-tasting liquors can also be concocted by adding several sprigs of tarragon, plus a mix of other herbs of one's choice, to a bottle of grappa, gin, or vodka, and left to macerate several weeks before straining and mixing with simple sugar syrup or mild honey, in equal or lesser amount, according to the strength desired.

# Southernwood

Also known as "old man," southernwood is a woody, stemmed, very pretty plant with a strong scent of camphor or lemon, depending on the variety. It contains high percentages of volatile oils camphor, eucalyptol, and absinthol, which are responsible for its aroma and its bitter, almost inedible taste. Despite this bitterness, southernwood is not poisonous and can be used in miniscule amounts to flavor such hearty dishes as beef or mutton stew.

Southernwood is more useful, however, as an insect and moth repellent, and can be used to very good effect in sachets for closets, drawers, and knitting baskets to protect wool and other fabrics.

Southernwood's delicate silvery foliage, so lovely in an herb garden, is often used in both dried and fresh flower arrangements, where it not only looks beautiful but also adds a fresh, brisk scent that lasts for weeks. Its leaves can be used in the bath for a soothing session of hydrotherapy that, due to the eucalyptol and camphor oils, also helps clear the sinuses. A strong antiseptic mouth rinse can be made by steeping its leaves in hot water, then letting it cool, and straining before use.

Old wives' tales say that a scalp tonic made from southernwood and rosemary will make hair grow back on balding heads or start a beard on a young man's face; hence southernwood's other folk name, "lad's love."

As with most Artemisias, southernwood flowers at the end of summer, if at all, with unattractive yellowish panicles. Propagation is by division, cuttings, or seed.

# Mugwort

Mugwort (*Artemisia vulgaris*), sometimes called old woman or sailor's tobacco, is the plant you have probably seen growing along the side of unkempt country roads or at the edges of overgrazed pastures, and thought it was a weed. It grows to about two feet in height, with coarser, larger, darker leaves than most other Artemisias, and thick, but not woody, purplish stems. If you rub its foliage, it gives off a spicy floral aroma, which can be attributed to its linalool content. Linalool is a terpenoid also found in lavender and bay laurel. Other volatile oils in mugwort are thujone, camphor, and eucalyptol.

For centuries mugwort has been used as a strewing herb, because of its pleasantly clean scent and antiseptic properties. In Chinese medicine it holds an important place as a cure for rheumatic aches, where it is used in moxicombustion. At certain acupuncture points, a wad of mugwort, called a *moxa*, is burnt upon the skin of the afflicted person to create a small burn scab, which apparently works to heal joint pains.

There is so much wild mugwort growing around where I live that I have never considered putting it in my herb garden, but one could easily plant it from seed. Mugwort blooms in late summer with brown panicles which then quickly go to seed—its main means of propagation. It gets its folk name sailor's tobacco because it can be dried and smoked in lieu of regular tobacco, although this is not recommended, because it contains thujone, a muscle convulsant. Its smoke will quickly clear the air of insects.

# Wormwood

*Artemisia absinthum* was made infamous because of its role as an ingredient in absinthe, the evil European liquor popular among artists in the late 1800s. Along with rue, wormwood is considered one of the bitterest of all herbs. Wormwood is mentioned in the book of Revelation, in the New Testament of the Christian Bible, as being the name of the star that signifies the end of the world!

The volatile oil absinthol is what gives wormwood its bitterness, but the plant also contains the terpene thujone. In large amounts and/or with prolonged use, thujone can have unpleasant and dangerous effects on human beings, including insomnia, anxiety, muscle spasms, convulsions, and eventually death, but wormwood contains only a small amount of this particular terpene, which, when steeped for use in alcoholic beverages, is generally considered safe in moderation. Wormwood is used in other beverages besides absinthe, including vermouth, bitters, Moroccan mint tea, and the Italian digestive genepì.

Previous to the days of absinthe, or "The Green Fairy," wormwood's main claim to fame was as a vermifuge, and hence its name. It is also an effective insect repellent and useful strewing herb. One of wormwood's sesquiterpene lactones, artemisinin, has been used in Chinese medicine since 200 BC for its anti-malarial function. Only in 1972 did medical scientists "prove" that artemisinin does indeed kill the bacteria that causes malaria.

Because of wormwood's extremely bitter taste, no one would likely want to eat it, which is fine because its foliage is considered unsafe for human consumption. However, the leaves of the plant can be steeped in boiled water to make a strong tea in which to soak compresses. These will relieve joint pain due to arthritis, rheumatism, or mild athletic injury. A warm footbath with several sprigs of wormwood and a tablespoon of coarse sea salt added will relieve tired, sore feet, with the additional bonus of the plant's antifungal and antiseptic properties thrown in.

Wormwood thrives in poor, dry soil, in full sun. It is propagated by cuttings, division, or seed, but be aware that, because of its high content of absinthin oil, which is toxic to most other plants, nothing will grow close to it.

## Sagebrush

*Artemisia tridentata* is also known as big sage, black sage, or sacred sage, and is native to the western plains of the United States. Despite its name, it is not a member of the sage genus! It is a gray-leaved, woody-stemmed bush or small tree, and, like other Artemisias, thrives in dry soil. Strongly aromatic, and redolent of actual sage (*Salvia officinalis*), it contains the terpenes eucalyptol, thujone, camphor, and linalool.

Although its taste is unpleasantly bitter, cattle and other ruminants left for long periods on the plains of the United States and Canada's Great Basin will graze on it, lacking anything better. The highly antiseptic terpene oils then kill the natural bacteria in these animals' rumen, which eventually leads to death.

Sagebrush is a strong vermifuge, and was used by Native Americans for that purpose, as well as in cleansing and purifying rituals and as an insect repellent. Compresses were soaked in sagebrush tea and used to treat infections.

Sagebrush's yellow blossom at the end of summer is Nevada's state flower, as the plant is the primary vegetation of that part of the United States.

## Using Artemisias in the Garden

Many people like to plant species of *Artemisia* in moon gardens because of their genus name, and why not? These beautiful, often silvery or lacy-leaved perennial plants look splendid under the light of the full moon, and make an excellent backdrop or neighbor to night-blooming flowers such as sweet-smelling white, pink, or red tobacco (*Nicotiana alata*), delicate climbing white moonflower (*Ipomea alba*), white or violet fragrant four o'clocks (*Mirabilis jalapa*), the majestic yellow scented evening primrose (*Oenothera biennis*), night-blooming white lilies, and perfumed white jasmine (*Jasminum*).

If you choose to plant Artemisias in your herb garden, give them a section all to themselves, where their potent terpenes will not inhibit other herbs' growth. Make sure they have plenty of space to spread, and full sun, and they will flourish with little or no nurturing. At the end of summer, after they've finished blooming, they will likely be very tall—as high as two or two and a half feet. Their tops will begin to look tangled, dry, or just plain ratty. Look at the base of the plant and you'll see the new, fresh green foliage already beginning to grow in. This is the time to cut down all the old growth. That new little bunch of green at the base will overwinter easily, in temperatures as low as –30° F. In the early spring, divide the plants for your own garden or for someone else's, and be ready for another perennial growing season of Artemisias.

# Herbal Philosophy

### ≈ by Calantirniel ≈

How many of you have heard offhand comments from people that "herbs do not work," only to discover they never really tried herbs properly? Most herbals on the market are written for the layperson, and unfortunately lack a deeper background on how to integrate herbs into our nutrition and health regimens. This requires an entirely different and expanded, holistic viewpoint rather than the compartmentalized, specialist-oriented lens through which we usually examine the world in our current culture. And to be fair, even the herbals that are written with proper background of herbs could be consulted only as a reference where the user looks up the

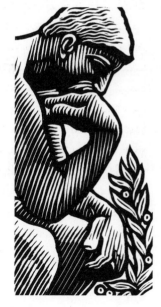

herb or symptoms in the index and never reads the important introductory material in the front of the book.

Here is one example of a person with a negative opinion of herbs based on misinformation. This man had a headache, so he Google-searched "herbs for headache" and discovered feverfew at the top of the list, since it is popularly marketed for this purpose; but he failed to research the underlying cause of his headache. Upon purchasing capsules at the grocery, he took them according to the label. They did not work to resolve the headache, because unbeknownst to him, feverfew was not the right herb for his headache. Yet based on this one stand-alone experience, he came to the drastic and rather irrational conclusion that all herbs do not work for any health problems!

While this may seem like an isolated incident, there are indeed many people who have had similar experiences. Since people are extremely busy with their lives nowadays, it is discouraging to know that many people do not have the drive or the time to truly discover this wonderful healing modality. What is also sad is that people often just want the symptoms of pain to go away without regard for the method through which this would be accomplished. Prescription and over-the-counter drugs have a suppressive effect on the body (antibiotics being the only exception, and they have their own problems) and do not solve the underlying issue. However, the underlying issue is never acknowledged—only the fact that the pain has temporarily left. But as we all know, there comes a point where suppression of symptoms doesn't work anymore and there are likely even newer problems that have become rather evident, and quite persistent.

We are taught that pain is bad, when technically it is at times the only way our body can communicate with us that something is out of balance. We need to retrain ourselves to be thankful for the pain experience (as unpleasant as it is) rather than suppress it. We instead need to find a way to correct the underlying issue that is responsible for the pain signal in the first place.

When the body has what it needs, it uses everything in balance to create homeostasis, or sustained health. When thrown out of balance for any reason, the body will use its vital life force in ways hard for us to imagine to re-create that level of homeostasis. This beautiful process is what could be termed *vitalism*, and the vitalistic approach for healing is to give the body what it needs and allow it in all its wisdom to heal on its own. So what does the body need?

Basically, what the body needs may be nutritional, or it may facilitate the body to properly eliminate. Herbs support this vitalistic process because plants are entirely better chemists than we are. Should this be a surprise? Not really, when we think about how much longer plants have been on the earth than we have! They need to remain rooted in soil and cannot move to get away from predators, and in turn they have developed some amazing living chemistry. We can choose to build a relationship with the gifts of the plant kingdom to inspire life and health on all levels. How can we do this?

First, we develop a relationship with our bodies, where communication (in the form of feelings) can relay important information about what the body needs. Often, the state of disease (that is, the lack of ease) can impart lessons for us to learn, and we can implement spiritual or energy work here if desired. This can be quite a process on its own, especially if conditions are considered hereditary.

Then, we need to learn about, and deeply respect, members of the plant kingdom (and the fungi kingdom, since many healers are also here). While some plants are quite poisonous, other plants are friendly for humans and are even considered food. And some plants are in between, providing strong medicine when it is needed that moves the body toward a healing response. With a proper approach, harvesting, preparation, and consumption, we can achieve true healing that addresses and corrects the underlying issues.

Herbalists spend much time studying known plant properties as well as developing relationships with the plants themselves so they know the right herb (or herbal combination) to address each of the areas of the body that need attention—and this also means gaining a working knowledge of illness in general, with all its various expressions. They also need to develop a relationship with the person for whom the herbal protocol is intended, since everyone is different (not unlike the plants).

To reframe this idea, pretend you are an owner of a business who needs to fill a position. You could hire a person to do the job, or you could purchase a robot that does only a specific task. While that particular task may be perfectly done by the robot, it may not be cost-effective since the company's needs will change and shift over time, rendering the robot inefficient in the long run. A person, on the other hand, can not only learn new things when placed in a new environment, but can adapt and possibly even figure out better solutions to reach the goal. Putting a different person in the position means different talents will be brought to the table. This new person could be more efficient in some ways, whereas the prior person was better in other ways.

To explain: the company is your body, its goal of success is in essence creating health and vitality, and the job opening is where the company isn't running so well (i.e., illness). Implementing an herb is similar to hiring a person, and using a prescription or over-the-counter medication is likened to hiring a robot that does only one task. To take this example even further, plants do have a well-documented history of efficacy (which we will call their resumé), but if asked by the body to do something different, it is possible for the plant to "stretch" its abilities in new ways and areas, and while it may never be better than another plant at a particular action, it seems that available plants often "make do" toward bringing the body to a healthier place. Medications can never change their action—and in fact are actually designed to force a particular action whether it is needed or not. You can easily see how some herbs can work together for an even better result, where mixing medications could cause more problems.

If you are using medications for chronic conditions and wish to switch to herbs in your health protocol, it is advisable to work with a knowledgeable team to see how this can be accomplished with the least distress possible. The actions of herbs work very differently, and the mixed messages can make the body go into shock. With some medications, like blood thinners and blood pressure drugs, it is imperative to very closely monitor vital signs during the transition.

So, let's go back to the example of the man who decided to use feverfew for his headache, but this time he has a better understanding of how herbs work. Perhaps when he Google-searches "herbs for headaches," he may discover there are many underlying causes of headaches, each of which may require a different herbal protocol. For example, it is surprising how many people with headaches find relief when they use herbs that gently expel the colon; constipation is one of the top causes of headaches, and hydration with good drinking water can also go a long way toward headache relief. Another cause (especially for females) is hormone imbalance, and often herbs that clear and renourish the liver will help immensely. If a headache is a result of having the flu, there are herbs that will quiet the nerves and soothe the circulatory system while assisting the body in ridding itself of the invading virus and strengthening the immune system. Still, a headache could have been caused by an old or new head injury, which requires herbs that clear the blood and may even be specific to the head area.

Once the underlying cause of a health issue is being addressed, herbs that can accommodate these main actions can be combined with other herbs for nutritional support as well as herbs that calm the nerves, lessening the pain response. If the cause is not clear, think about the problems you started having first and you may find clues. If this still doesn't help, consult an herbalist or other knowledgeable holistic health care provider to help untangle the body's signals and find the perfect herbal program for you. I hope this article helps you achieve a deeper level of health and vitality!

## Resources

Wood, Matthew. *The Earthwise Herbal: A Complete Guide to New World Medicinal Plants.* Berkeley, CA: North Atlantic Books, 2009.

———. *The Earthwise Herbal: A Complete Guide to Old World Medicinal Plants.* Berkeley, CA: North Atlantic Books, 2008.

Wood, Matthew. *Vitalism: The History of Herbalism, Homeopathy and Flower Essences*. Second Edition. Berkeley, CA: North Atlantic Books, 2005.

## Internet Resources

Many herbal resources can be found here: *The AstroHerbalist, AarTiana*, http://astroherbalist.com.

# The Numerology of Plants

∗ by Kelly Proudfoot ∗

Numerology has long been considered the key to all things in
the universe. The ancients believed
that everything could be understood
through the numerological components that are inherently contained
in people, objects, events, and even
animals and plants. Along with planetary influences, numerology is an
interesting guide to understanding
the meaning of life and the things
within it.

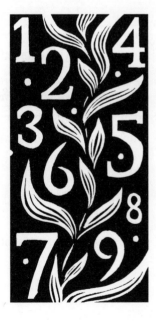

Nicholas Culpeper, who is famous
for his work—notably his book the
*Complete Herbal*, published in 1653—
believed in working with the planetary
influences involved with the propagation, growing, harvesting, and use of

herbs and plants. A lot of modern-day herbalists and gardeners take into consideration the phases of the moon when planting and tending their gardens, whether the gardens are used to produce vegetables, fruits, and herbs or are just for ornamental use.

The properties of herbs and plants can be understood from a numerological perspective, especially when you want to align those properties with a particular purpose. Whether it be because you want a certain outcome or certain energies involved in the creation of herbal sachets or mojo bags, potpourris, oils, or teas, numerology enhances the understanding of their properties.

I admit that it might seem odd to apply numerology to plants. When I've tried in the past to research correspondences regarding herbs and numerology, I've often hit brick walls. But as a numerologist and a Hedgewitch who has her own herbal garden and uses herbs and plants in ritual, I found I had the information right at my fingertips. Using plants and herbs can be complex when determining the correspondences for the desired purpose. There are scores of books on the properties of herbs, some of which are good; but it can be daunting to break it all down even further and to understand rudimentary things such as planetary and numerological influences.

You don't have to be an expert on numerology to utilize the numerological aspects of herbs and plants. Using the base numbers, 1–9, and understanding the basic meaning of each number is enough to be able to plan what herbs and plants are to be used for any purpose.

Before we look at the basic meanings of each number, let's look at how to calculate your Personality and Destiny numbers. These are the two basic numbers that you will use most often.

When using numerology, I use only the base numbers, 1–9. All numbers can be reduced to a single digit, and all numbers above 9 are formed using the base numbers. This is the way I was taught and the way that has proven to be the most correct and exact for me. If you like using Master numbers such as 11 or 22, that's fine if it works for you. But I find it's best to keep things pure and simple.

To calculate your Personality number, reduce the day of your birth to a single digit, unless it's already a single digit, such as a 2. So if you were born on the 23rd of the month, then just add 2 and 3 together to make 5.

To calculate your Destiny (or Life Path) number, total the numbers in your whole birth date. For example, September 5, 1966, becomes 9 + 5 + 1 + 9 + 6 + 6 = 36 = 3 + 6 = 9. Always reduce to a single digit.

## The Numerology of Plants

The first chart given here lists the keywords, planet, and color associated with each base number. The second chart lists the herbs, plants, and purposes associated with each base number.

There are many other attributes for each number, but in order to keep things simple I've included just the main properties. When choosing herbs and plants for particular purposes from a numerological perspective, these charts will help you get on the right path.

| Base Number | Keywords | Planet | Color |
|---|---|---|---|
| 1 | Creation, beginnings, independence | Sun | Yellow |
| 2 | Balance, unity, intuition | Moon | White |
| 3 | Expression, vision, inspiration | Jupiter | Orange |
| 4 | Structure, discipline, restrictions | Saturn | Black |
| 5 | Freedom, change, intellect | Mercury | Green |
| 6 | Responsibility, love, healing | Venus | Pink |
| 7 | Spirituality, learning, analysis | Neptune | Purple |
| 8 | Wealth, ego, ambition | Mars | Red |
| 9 | Universal consciousness, completion, compassion | Pluto | Navy blue |

Chart 1: Keywords, planet, and color associated with each base number.

Chart 2 *(opposite page)*: Herbs, plants, and purposes associated with each base number.

| Base Number | Herbs/Plants | Purpose |
|---|---|---|
| 1 | Cinnamon, oak, bay, rosemary, frankincense, orange | To gain independence |
| 2 | Lemon, cucumber, gardenia, myrrh, poppy, willow | To promote unity |
| 3 | Sage, nutmeg, anise, cinquefoil, clove, honeysuckle | To strengthen communication |
| 4 | Solomon's seal, ivy, cypress, poplar, skullcap, beech | To ensure stability and security |
| 5 | Almond, mint, mandrake, lavender, fern, caraway | To gain freedom |
| 6 | Catnip, apple, coltsfoot, elder, blackberry, peach | To gain love and peace |
| 7 | Bodhi, angelica, sandalwood, valerian, mugwort, thyme | To promote second sight |
| 8 | Chili, cumin, damiana, garlic, peppermint, galangal | To attain prosperity and success |
| 9 | Ash, mulberry, Job's tears, mustard, iris, sunflower | To develop compassion and wisdom |

In order to manifest any of the energies you wish to emulate, choose three to five herbs/plants for the particular number and carry in a mojo bag of the related color. You might also like to experiment with things such as the number of petals on a flower or the number of leaves. Think about the color of the herb/plant and see if that corresponds to its numerological properties. Take into consideration the season or blooming time for the plant. What planetary hour does it correspond to?

Using numerology is a great way to personalize your workings and align the properties of herbs and plants with any purpose.

# A Dinosaur in Your Backyard: Meet the Horsetail

### ⪼ Susan Pesznecker ⪻

Every spring, without fail, my yard is overrun by dinosaurs: greenish brown, scaly dinosaurs that run in dense tribes and seem to appear everywhere I look. Has my land been invaded by sauropods? Nope. My dinosaurs go by the name of *Equisetum*: the common horsetail.

The genus *Equisetum*, comprising plants known as horsetails or horsetail ferns (although they are not ferns at all), is, in fact, a living fossil that is more or less unchanged from *Equisetum* species that flourished 400 million years ago in the Paleozoic era. It's a fascinating plant with a rich ethnographic history and medicinal uses as well.

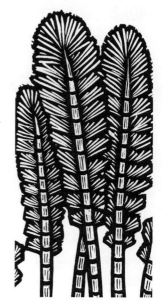

The horsetail probably gets its common name from its bushy tail–like appearance. Other folk names include bottle-brush, Dutch rush, horse willow, paddock pipes, pewterwort, puzzlegrass, scouring rush, shave grass, snake grass, and toad pipe, each reflecting either the horsetail's appearance or a common use. Its scientific names comes from the Latin *equis* ("horse") + *seta* ("bristle"), again conjuring up that image of the bushy or brushy tail.

In Paleozoic times the horsetail was a tree that could reach 80 to 100 feet; today's version is a bushy perennial that might reach 3 to 4 feet, depending on species and local conditions. Horsetail is found on every continent but Antarctica, but favors damp, lowland locales with loose soil and good drainage. In warm climates it thrives year round, while in colder climes it dies back in winter and reemerges each spring. It's a perennial and spreads by deep, somewhat brittle rhizomes, making it very difficult to dig out and eradicate. (Translation: If you miss or break off a one-inch section of rhizome, a new plant will grow from it!) The plant is not sensitive to traditional herbicides. In some locations it is classified as a nuisance weed, and in others (including my own Oregon) it's considered a noxious plant.

The typical horsetail plant has between one and five stems, each with a number of brush-like "leaves" that don't look like leaves at all. The stems are hollow and ridged and connected by "joints" that can be pulled apart and reassembled. The plants reproduce through spore-bearing structures on the tips of some stems. Horsetail is rich in silica; as the plant matures and then begins to dry and fade, the silica crystals within the desiccating plant make it feel rough and scratchy.

Medicinally, the aerial parts of the common field horsetail (*E. arvense*) are used in a number of medicinal treatments. Dioscorides noted horsetail's value in staunching bleeding and treating wounds, and today's herbalists know that a simmered decoction of horsetail and water is effective for treating skin irritations, small wounds, and inflamed gums. An infusion of fresh or dried leaves is useful for lung problems, stomach ulcers, and menstrual problems, and juice taken from the fresh plant acts as a diuretic and treats anemia, edema, and bladder infections. Recent research has proven horsetail's antioxidant nature and has suggested it—because of its high silica content—as a possible treatment for osteoporosis due to silica's role in regenerating connective tissue.

Note, however, that horsetail isn't innocuous. It may bind with thiamine (vitamin B1), causing levels of the vitamin to drop below normal. Because the plant contains trace amounts of nicotine, it should not be used to treat children. If taken internally, exacting recommendations must be followed to avoid toxicity. Only *E. arvense* should be used medicinally; other species are toxic.

Ethnographically, horsetail had a number of practical uses. Because of its high silica levels and abrasive feel, ancient peoples used it to scour cooking vessels; hence the folk name "scouring rush." The young stems may be harvested and eaten raw or may be steamed and eaten like a type of spring asparagus. Older stems are dried and powdered to make a thickening agent for stews and soups. The young green leaves make a green dye, and some woodworkers today still use dried horsetail plants as a type of sandpaper for fine polishing of wood projects. The writer and biologist Dr. Jim Pojar also tells of the plant's use as a tool in analyzing the amount of gold in a liquid solution, as the plants take up gold quickly and at a predictable rate.

The plant may have mathematical relevance, too. It's been suggested that Scottish mathematician John Napier, when observing the arrangement of horsetail's nodes and whorls, may have used his observations to identify and describe the idea of logarithms. Or perhaps you're looking for a more romantic tale: how about the one that tells of using horsetail stems to create fairy whistles for calling the fae folk?

Horsetail poses a bit of a challenge for those who find it in their gardens (as I do), for it spreads voraciously by rhizome, posing interesting gardening challenges. If you simply yank it out of the ground—and it does come up easily—you break the rhizome; now, instead of one plant, you'll have two. Digging the rhizome is effective but painstaking, and again, if you leave any broken rootstalk, more plants will appear. The plant is sensitive to certain chemical herbicides, but even so may be almost impossible to eradicate. My means of dealing with horsetail is to cut it or pull it up as I find it. I toss it onto the lawn, where my mulching mower pulverizes it and gives its nutrients and minerals back to the soil. Sometimes I just toss it into the compost pile.

To harvest horsetail, cut the stems during summer and air-dry. Store in jars in a cool, light-tight cupboard for up to 1 to 2 years.

If you have a farm and feed large animals, be wary: horsetail is poisonous or toxic to livestock and must not be harvested with the hay cutting.

# Sources

"Horsetail." *University of Maryland Medical Center.* Reviewed March 5, 2011. http://www.umm.edu/altmed/articles /horsetail-000257.htm.

Pojar, Jim. *Plants of the Pacific Northwest Coast: Washington, Oregon, British Columbia & Alaska.* Auburn, WA: Lone Pine, 2004.

Sacks, Oliver. "Field Trip: Hunting Horsetails." *The New Yorker.* August 2011.

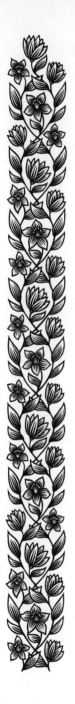

# Moon Signs, Phases, and Tables

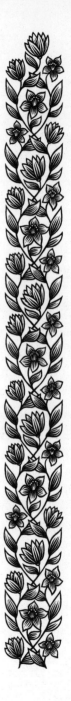

# The Quarters and Signs
# of the Moon

Everyone has seen the moon wax and wane through a period of approximately 29½ days. This circuit from new moon to full moon and back again is called the lunation cycle. The cycle is divided into parts called quarters or phases. There are several methods by which this can be done, and the system used in the *Herbal Almanac* may not correspond to those used in other almanacs.

## The Quarters

### First Quarter

The first quarter begins at the new moon, when the sun and moon are in the same place, or conjunct. (This means the sun and moon are in the same degree of the same sign.) The moon is not visible at first, since it rises at the same time as the sun. The new moon is the time of new beginnings of projects that favor growth, externalization of activities, and the growth of ideas. The first quarter is the time of germination, emergence, beginnings, and outwardly directed activity.

### Second Quarter

The second quarter begins halfway between the new moon and the full moon, when the sun and moon are at a right angle, or a 90° square, to each other. This half moon rises around noon and sets around midnight, so it can be seen in the western sky during the first half of the night. The second quarter is the time of growth and articulation of things that already exist.

## Third Quarter

The third quarter begins at the full moon, when the sun and moon are opposite one another and the full light of the sun can shine on the full sphere of the moon. The round moon can be seen rising in the east at sunset, then rising a little later each evening. The full moon stands for illumination, fulfillment, culmination, completion, drawing inward, unrest, emotional expressions, and hasty actions leading to failure. The third quarter is a time of maturity, fruition, and the assumption of the full form of expression.

## Fourth Quarter

The fourth quarter begins about halfway between the full moon and the new moon, when the sun and moon are again at a right angle, or a 90° square, to each other. This decreasing moon rises at midnight and can be seen in the east during the last half of the night, reaching the overhead position just about as the sun rises. The fourth quarter is a time of disintegration and drawing back for reorganization and reflection.

# The Signs

## Moon in Aries

Moon in Aries is good for starting things and initiating change, but actions may lack staying power. Activities requiring assertiveness and courage are favored. Things occur rapidly but also quickly pass.

## Moon in Taurus

Things begun when the moon is in Taurus last the longest and tend to increase in value. This is a good time for any activity that requires patience, practicality, and perseverance. Things begun now also tend to become habitual and hard to alter.

## Moon in Gemini

Moon in Gemini is a good time to exchange ideas, meet with people, or be in situations that require versatility and quick thinking. Things begun now are easily changed by outside influences.

## Moon in Cancer

Moon in Cancer is a good time to grow things. It stimulates emotional rapport between people and is a good time to build personal friendships, though people may be more emotional and moody than usual.

## Moon in Leo

Moon in Leo is a good time for public appearances, showmanship, being seen, entertaining, drama, recreation, and happy pursuits. People may be overly concerned with praise and subject to flattery.

## Moon in Virgo

Moon in Virgo is good for any task that requires close attention to detail and careful analysis of information. There is a focus on health, hygiene, and daily schedules. Watch for a tendency to overdo and overwork.

## Moon in Libra

Moon in Libra is a good time to form partnerships of any kind and to negotiate. It discourages spontaneous initiative, so working with a partner is essential. Artistic work and teamwork are highlighted.

## Moon in Scorpio

Moon in Scorpio increases awareness of psychic power and favors any activity that requires intensity and focus. This is a good time to conduct research and to end connections thoroughly. There is a tendency to manipulate.

## Moon in Sagittarius

Moon in Sagittarius is good for any activity that requires honesty, candor, imagination, and confidence in the flow of life. This is a good time to tackle things that need improvement, but watch out for a tendency to proselytize.

## Moon in Capricorn

Moon in Capricorn increases awareness of the need for structure, discipline, and patience. This is a good time to set goals and plan for the future. Those in authority may be insensitive at this time.

## Moon in Aquarius

Moon in Aquarius favors activities that are unique and individualistic and that concern society as a whole. This is a good time to pursue humanitarian efforts and to identify improvements that can be made. People may be more intellectual than emotional under this influence.

## Moon in Pisces

Moon in Pisces is a good time for any kind of introspective, philanthropic, meditative, psychic, or artistic work. At this time personal boundaries may be blurred, and people may be prone to seeing what they want to see rather than what is really there.

# January Moon Table

| Date | Sign | Element | Nature | Phase |
|---|---|---|---|---|
| 1 Tue 12:35 pm | Virgo | Earth | Barren | 3rd |
| 2 Wed | Virgo | Earth | Barren | 3rd |
| 3 Thu 8:11 pm | Libra | Air | Semi-fruitful | 3rd |
| 4 Fri | Libra | Air | Semi-fruitful | 4th 10:58 pm |
| 5 Sat | Libra | Air | Semi-fruitful | 4th |
| 6 Sun 1:09 am | Scorpio | Water | Fruitful | 4th |
| 7 Mon | Scorpio | Water | Fruitful | 4th |
| 8 Tue 3:28 am | Sagittarius | Fire | Barren | 4th |
| 9 Wed | Sagittarius | Fire | Barren | 4th |
| 10 Thu 3:54 am | Capricorn | Earth | Semi-fruitful | 4th |
| 11 Fri | Capricorn | Earth | Semi-fruitful | New 2:44 pm |
| 12 Sat 4:01 am | Aquarius | Air | Barren | 1st |
| 13 Sun | Aquarius | Air | Barren | 1st |
| 14 Mon 5:49 am | Pisces | Water | Fruitful | 1st |
| 15 Tue | Pisces | Water | Fruitful | 1st |
| 16 Wed 11:07 am | Aries | Fire | Barren | 1st |
| 17 Thu | Aries | Fire | Barren | 1st |
| 18 Fri 8:36 pm | Taurus | Earth | Semi-fruitful | 2nd 6:45 pm |
| 19 Sat | Taurus | Earth | Semi-fruitful | 2nd |
| 20 Sun | Taurus | Earth | Semi-fruitful | 2nd |
| 21 Mon 9:04 am | Gemini | Air | Barren | 2nd |
| 22 Tue | Gemini | Air | Barren | 2nd |
| 23 Wed 10:00 pm | Cancer | Water | Fruitful | 2nd |
| 24 Thu | Cancer | Water | Fruitful | 2nd |
| 25 Fri | Cancer | Water | Fruitful | 2nd |
| 26 Sat 9:20 am | Leo | Fire | Barren | Full 11:38 pm |
| 27 Sun | Leo | Fire | Barren | 3rd |
| 28 Mon 6:27 pm | Virgo | Earth | Barren | 3rd |
| 29 Tue | Virgo | Earth | Barren | 3rd |
| 30 Wed | Virgo | Earth | Barren | 3rd |
| 31 Thu 1:36 am | Libra | Air | Semi-fruitful | 3rd |

# February Moon Table

| Date | Sign | Element | Nature | Phase |
|------|------|---------|--------|-------|
| 1 Fri | Libra | Air | Semi-fruitful | 3rd |
| 2 Sat 7:02 am | Scorpio | Water | Fruitful | 3rd |
| 3 Sun | Scorpio | Water | Fruitful | 4th 8:56 am |
| 4 Mon 10:45 am | Sagittarius | Fire | Barren | 4th |
| 5 Tue | Sagittarius | Fire | Barren | 4th |
| 6 Wed 12:55 pm | Capricorn | Earth | Semi-fruitful | 4th |
| 7 Thu | Capricorn | Earth | Semi-fruitful | 4th |
| 8 Fri 2:16 pm | Aquarius | Air | Barren | 4th |
| 9 Sat | Aquarius | Air | Barren | 4th |
| 10 Sun 4:20 pm | Pisces | Water | Fruitful | New 2:20 am |
| 11 Mon | Pisces | Water | Fruitful | 1st |
| 12 Tue 8:51 pm | Aries | Fire | Barren | 1st |
| 13 Wed | Aries | Fire | Barren | 1st |
| 14 Thu | Aries | Fire | Barren | 1st |
| 15 Fri 5:08 am | Taurus | Earth | Semi-fruitful | 1st |
| 16 Sat | Taurus | Earth | Semi-fruitful | 1st |
| 17 Sun 4:50 pm | Gemini | Air | Barren | 2nd 3:31 pm |
| 18 Mon | Gemini | Air | Barren | 2nd |
| 19 Tue | Gemini | Air | Barren | 2nd |
| 20 Wed 5:45 am | Cancer | Water | Fruitful | 2nd |
| 21 Thu | Cancer | Water | Fruitful | 2nd |
| 22 Fri 5:12 pm | Leo | Fire | Barren | 2nd |
| 23 Sat | Leo | Fire | Barren | 2nd |
| 24 Sun | Leo | Fire | Barren | 2nd |
| 25 Mon 1:52 am | Virgo | Earth | Barren | Full 3:26 pm |
| 26 Tue | Virgo | Earth | Barren | 3rd |
| 27 Wed 8:02 am | Libra | Air | Semi-fruitful | 3rd |
| 28 Thu | Libra | Air | Semi-fruitful | 3rd |

*Times are in Eastern Time.*

# March Moon Table

| Date | Sign | Element | Nature | Phase |
|------|------|---------|--------|-------|
| 1 Fri 12:33 pm | Scorpio | Water | Fruitful | 3rd |
| 2 Sat | Scorpio | Water | Fruitful | 3rd |
| 3 Sun 4:11 pm | Sagittarius | Fire | Barren | 3rd |
| 4 Mon | Sagittarius | Fire | Barren | 4th 4:53 pm |
| 5 Tue 7:14 pm | Capricorn | Earth | Semi-fruitful | 4th |
| 6 Wed | Capricorn | Earth | Semi-fruitful | 4th |
| 7 Thu 10:01 pm | Aquarius | Air | Barren | 4th |
| 8 Fri | Aquarius | Air | Barren | 4th |
| 9 Sat | Aquarius | Air | Barren | 4th |
| 10 Sun 1:19 am | Pisces | Water | Fruitful | 4th |
| 11 Mon | Pisces | Water | Fruitful | New 3:51 pm |
| 12 Tue 7:17 am | Aries | Fire | Barren | 1st |
| 13 Wed | Aries | Fire | Barren | 1st |
| 14 Thu 3:08 pm | Taurus | Earth | Semi-fruitful | 1st |
| 15 Fri | Taurus | Earth | Semi-fruitful | 1st |
| 16 Sat | Taurus | Earth | Semi-fruitful | 1st |
| 17 Sun 2:09 am | Gemini | Air | Barren | 1st |
| 18 Mon | Gemini | Air | Barren | 1st |
| 19 Tue 2:55 pm | Cancer | Water | Fruitful | 2nd 1:27 pm |
| 20 Wed | Cancer | Water | Fruitful | 2nd |
| 21 Thu | Cancer | Water | Fruitful | 2nd |
| 22 Fri 2:50 am | Leo | Fire | Barren | 2nd |
| 23 Sat | Leo | Fire | Barren | 2nd |
| 24 Sun 11:49 am | Virgo | Earth | Barren | 2nd |
| 25 Mon | Virgo | Earth | Barren | 2nd |
| 26 Tue 5:32 pm | Libra | Air | Semi-fruitful | 2nd |
| 27 Wed | Libra | Air | Semi-fruitful | Full 5:27 am |
| 28 Thu 8:53 pm | Scorpio | Water | Fruitful | 3rd |
| 29 Fri | Scorpio | Water | Fruitful | 3rd |
| 30 Sat 11:13 pm | Sagittarius | Fire | Barren | 3rd |
| 31 Sun | Sagittarius | Fire | Barren | 3rd |

# April Moon Table

| Date | Sign | Element | Nature | Phase |
|------|------|---------|--------|-------|
| 1 Mon | Sagittarius | Fire | Barren | 3rd |
| 2 Tue 1:35 am | Capricorn | Earth | Semi-fruitful | 3rd |
| 3 Wed | Capricorn | Earth | Semi-fruitful | 4th 12:37 am |
| 4 Thu 4:41 am | Aquarius | Air | Barren | 4th |
| 5 Fri | Aquarius | Air | Barren | 4th |
| 6 Sat 9:00 am | Pisces | Water | Fruitful | 4th |
| 7 Sun | Pisces | Water | Fruitful | 4th |
| 8 Mon 3:02 pm | Aries | Fire | Barren | 4th |
| 9 Tue | Aries | Fire | Barren | 4th |
| 10 Wed 11:22 pm | Taurus | Earth | Semi-fruitful | New 5:35 am |
| 11 Thu | Taurus | Earth | Semi-fruitful | 1st |
| 12 Fri | Taurus | Earth | Semi-fruitful | 1st |
| 13 Sat 10:13 am | Gemini | Air | Barren | 1st |
| 14 Sun | Gemini | Air | Barren | 1st |
| 15 Mon 10:49 pm | Cancer | Water | Fruitful | 1st |
| 16 Tue | Cancer | Water | Fruitful | 1st |
| 17 Wed | Cancer | Water | Fruitful | 1st |
| 18 Thu 11:13 am | Leo | Fire | Barren | 2nd 8:31 am |
| 19 Fri | Leo | Fire | Barren | 2nd |
| 20 Sat 9:08 pm | Virgo | Earth | Barren | 2nd |
| 21 Sun | Virgo | Earth | Barren | 2nd |
| 22 Mon | Virgo | Earth | Barren | 2nd |
| 23 Tue 3:25 am | Libra | Air | Semi-fruitful | 2nd |
| 24 Wed | Libra | Air | Semi-fruitful | 2nd |
| 25 Thu 6:25 am | Scorpio | Water | Fruitful | Full 3:57 pm |
| 26 Fri | Scorpio | Water | Fruitful | 3rd |
| 27 Sat 7:32 am | Sagittarius | Fire | Barren | 3rd |
| 28 Sun | Sagittarius | Fire | Barren | 3rd |
| 29 Mon 8:21 am | Capricorn | Earth | Semi-fruitful | 3rd |
| 30 Tue | Capricorn | Earth | Semi-fruitful | 3rd |

*Times are in Eastern Time.*

# May Moon Table

| Date | Sign | Element | Nature | Phase |
|------|------|---------|--------|-------|
| 1 Wed 10:20 am | Aquarius | Air | Barren | 3rd |
| 2 Thu | Aquarius | Air | Barren | 4th 7:14 am |
| 3 Fri 2:25 pm | Pisces | Water | Fruitful | 4th |
| 4 Sat | Pisces | Water | Fruitful | 4th |
| 5 Sun 9:03 pm | Aries | Fire | Barren | 4th |
| 6 Mon | Aries | Fire | Barren | 4th |
| 7 Tue | Aries | Fire | Barren | 4th |
| 8 Wed 6:09 am | Taurus | Earth | Semi-fruitful | 4th |
| 9 Thu | Taurus | Earth | Semi-fruitful | New 8:28 pm |
| 10 Fri 5:21 pm | Gemini | Air | Barren | 1st |
| 11 Sat | Gemini | Air | Barren | 1st |
| 12 Sun | Gemini | Air | Barren | 1st |
| 13 Mon 5:57 am | Cancer | Water | Fruitful | 1st |
| 14 Tue | Cancer | Water | Fruitful | 1st |
| 15 Wed 6:38 pm | Leo | Fire | Barren | 1st |
| 16 Thu | Leo | Fire | Barren | 1st |
| 17 Fri | Leo | Fire | Barren | 1st |
| 18 Sat 5:33 am | Virgo | Earth | Barren | 2nd 12:35 am |
| 19 Sun | Virgo | Earth | Barren | 2nd |
| 20 Mon 1:07 pm | Libra | Air | Semi-fruitful | 2nd |
| 21 Tue | Libra | Air | Semi-fruitful | 2nd |
| 22 Wed 4:55 pm | Scorpio | Water | Fruitful | 2nd |
| 23 Thu | Scorpio | Water | Fruitful | 2nd |
| 24 Fri 5:49 pm | Sagittarius | Fire | Barren | 2nd |
| 25 Sat | Sagittarius | Fire | Barren | Full 12:25 am |
| 26 Sun 5:28 pm | Capricorn | Earth | Semi-fruitful | 3rd |
| 27 Mon | Capricorn | Earth | Semi-fruitful | 3rd |
| 28 Tue 5:48 pm | Aquarius | Air | Barren | 3rd |
| 29 Wed | Aquarius | Air | Barren | 3rd |
| 30 Thu 8:30 pm | Pisces | Water | Fruitful | 3rd |
| 31 Fri | Pisces | Water | Fruitful | 4th 2:58 pm |

# June Moon Table

| Date | Sign | Element | Nature | Phase |
|------|------|---------|--------|-------|
| 1 Sat | Pisces | Water | Fruitful | 4th |
| 2 Sun 2:33 am | Aries | Fire | Barren | 4th |
| 3 Mon | Aries | Fire | Barren | 4th |
| 4 Tue 11:53 am | Taurus | Earth | Semi-fruitful | 4th |
| 5 Wed | Taurus | Earth | Semi-fruitful | 4th |
| 6 Thu 11:32 pm | Gemini | Air | Barren | 4th |
| 7 Fri | Gemini | Air | Barren | 4th |
| 8 Sat | Gemini | Air | Barren | New 11:56 am |
| 9 Sun 12:16 pm | Cancer | Water | Fruitful | 1st |
| 10 Mon | Cancer | Water | Fruitful | 1st |
| 11 Tue | Cancer | Water | Fruitful | 1st |
| 12 Wed 12:58 am | Leo | Fire | Barren | 1st |
| 13 Thu | Leo | Fire | Barren | 1st |
| 14 Fri 12:26 pm | Virgo | Earth | Barren | 1st |
| 15 Sat | Virgo | Earth | Barren | 1st |
| 16 Sun 9:19 pm | Libra | Air | Semi-fruitful | 2nd 1:24 pm |
| 17 Mon | Libra | Air | Semi-fruitful | 2nd |
| 18 Tue | Libra | Air | Semi-fruitful | 2nd |
| 19 Wed 2:38 am | Scorpio | Water | Fruitful | 2nd |
| 20 Thu | Scorpio | Water | Fruitful | 2nd |
| 21 Fri 4:31 am | Sagittarius | Fire | Barren | 2nd |
| 22 Sat | Sagittarius | Fire | Barren | 2nd |
| 23 Sun 4:08 am | Capricorn | Earth | Semi-fruitful | Full 7:32 am |
| 24 Mon | Capricorn | Earth | Semi-fruitful | 3rd |
| 25 Tue 3:27 am | Aquarius | Air | Barren | 3rd |
| 26 Wed | Aquarius | Air | Barren | 3rd |
| 27 Thu 4:32 am | Pisces | Water | Fruitful | 3rd |
| 28 Fri | Pisces | Water | Fruitful | 3rd |
| 29 Sat 9:07 am | Aries | Fire | Barren | 3rd |
| 30 Sun | Aries | Fire | Barren | 4th 12:54 am |

*Times are in Eastern Time.*

# July Moon Table

| Date | Sign | Element | Nature | Phase |
|------|------|---------|--------|-------|
| 1 Mon 5:43 pm | Taurus | Earth | Semi-fruitful | 4th |
| 2 Tue | Taurus | Earth | Semi-fruitful | 4th |
| 3 Wed | Taurus | Earth | Semi-fruitful | 4th |
| 4 Thu 5:21 am | Gemini | Air | Barren | 4th |
| 5 Fri | Gemini | Air | Barren | 4th |
| 6 Sat 6:14 pm | Cancer | Water | Fruitful | 4th |
| 7 Sun | Cancer | Water | Fruitful | 4th |
| 8 Mon | Cancer | Water | Fruitful | New 3:14 am |
| 9 Tue 6:48 am | Leo | Fire | Barren | 1st |
| 10 Wed | Leo | Fire | Barren | 1st |
| 11 Thu 6:12 pm | Virgo | Earth | Barren | 1st |
| 12 Fri | Virgo | Earth | Barren | 1st |
| 13 Sat | Virgo | Earth | Barren | 1st |
| 14 Sun 3:41 am | Libra | Air | Semi-fruitful | 1st |
| 15 Mon | Libra | Air | Semi-fruitful | 2nd 11:18 pm |
| 16 Tue 10:24 am | Scorpio | Water | Fruitful | 2nd |
| 17 Wed | Scorpio | Water | Fruitful | 2nd |
| 18 Thu 1:54 pm | Sagittarius | Fire | Barren | 2nd |
| 19 Fri | Sagittarius | Fire | Barren | 2nd |
| 20 Sat 2:39 pm | Capricorn | Earth | Semi-fruitful | 2nd |
| 21 Sun | Capricorn | Earth | Semi-fruitful | 2nd |
| 22 Mon 2:07 pm | Aquarius | Air | Barren | Full 2:16 pm |
| 23 Tue | Aquarius | Air | Barren | 3rd |
| 24 Wed 2:22 pm | Pisces | Water | Fruitful | 3rd |
| 25 Thu | Pisces | Water | Fruitful | 3rd |
| 26 Fri 5:29 pm | Aries | Fire | Barren | 3rd |
| 27 Sat | Aries | Fire | Barren | 3rd |
| 28 Sun | Aries | Fire | Barren | 3rd |
| 29 Mon 12:43 am | Taurus | Earth | Semi-fruitful | 4th 1:43 pm |
| 30 Tue | Taurus | Earth | Semi-fruitful | 4th |
| 31 Wed 11:42 am | Gemini | Air | Barren | 4th |

# August Moon Table

| Date | Sign | Element | Nature | Phase |
|------|------|---------|--------|-------|
| 1 Thu | Gemini | Air | Barren | 4th |
| 2 Fri | Gemini | Air | Barren | 4th |
| 3 Sat 12:29 am | Cancer | Water | Fruitful | 4th |
| 4 Sun | Cancer | Water | Fruitful | 4th |
| 5 Mon 12:58 pm | Leo | Fire | Barren | 4th |
| 6 Tue | Leo | Fire | Barren | New 5:51 pm |
| 7 Wed 11:57 pm | Virgo | Earth | Barren | 1st |
| 8 Thu | Virgo | Earth | Barren | 1st |
| 9 Fri | Virgo | Earth | Barren | 1st |
| 10 Sat 9:08 am | Libra | Air | Semi-fruitful | 1st |
| 11 Sun | Libra | Air | Semi-fruitful | 1st |
| 12 Mon 4:18 pm | Scorpio | Water | Fruitful | 1st |
| 13 Tue | Scorpio | Water | Fruitful | 1st |
| 14 Wed 9:04 pm | Sagittarius | Fire | Barren | 2nd 6:56 am |
| 15 Thu | Sagittarius | Fire | Barren | 2nd |
| 16 Fri 11:25 pm | Capricorn | Earth | Semi-fruitful | 2nd |
| 17 Sat | Capricorn | Earth | Semi-fruitful | 2nd |
| 18 Sun | Capricorn | Earth | Semi-fruitful | 2nd |
| 19 Mon 12:07 am | Aquarius | Air | Barren | 2nd |
| 20 Tue | Aquarius | Air | Barren | Full 9:45 pm |
| 21 Wed 12:43 am | Pisces | Water | Fruitful | 3rd |
| 22 Thu | Pisces | Water | Fruitful | 3rd |
| 23 Fri 3:13 am | Aries | Fire | Barren | 3rd |
| 24 Sat | Aries | Fire | Barren | 3rd |
| 25 Sun 9:13 am | Taurus | Earth | Semi-fruitful | 3rd |
| 26 Mon | Taurus | Earth | Semi-fruitful | 3rd |
| 27 Tue 7:08 pm | Gemini | Air | Barren | 3rd |
| 28 Wed | Gemini | Air | Barren | 4th 5:35 am |
| 29 Thu | Gemini | Air | Barren | 4th |
| 30 Fri 7:33 am | Cancer | Water | Fruitful | 4th |
| 31 Sat | Cancer | Water | Fruitful | 4th |

*Times are in Eastern Time.*

# September Moon Table

| Date | Sign | Element | Nature | Phase |
|------|------|---------|--------|-------|
| 1 Sun 8:01 pm | Leo | Fire | Barren | 4th |
| 2 Mon | Leo | Fire | Barren | 4th |
| 3 Tue | Leo | Fire | Barren | 4th |
| 4 Wed 6:43 am | Virgo | Earth | Barren | 4th |
| 5 Thu | Virgo | Earth | Barren | New 7:36 am |
| 6 Fri 3:12 pm | Libra | Air | Semi-fruitful | 1st |
| 7 Sat | Libra | Air | Semi-fruitful | 1st |
| 8 Sun 9:44 pm | Scorpio | Water | Fruitful | 1st |
| 9 Mon | Scorpio | Water | Fruitful | 1st |
| 10 Tue | Scorpio | Water | Fruitful | 1st |
| 11 Wed 2:36 am | Sagittarius | Fire | Barren | 1st |
| 12 Thu | Sagittarius | Fire | Barren | 2nd 1:08 pm |
| 13 Fri 5:56 am | Capricorn | Earth | Semi-fruitful | 2nd |
| 14 Sat | Capricorn | Earth | Semi-fruitful | 2nd |
| 15 Sun 8:05 am | Aquarius | Air | Barren | 2nd |
| 16 Mon | Aquarius | Air | Barren | 2nd |
| 17 Tue 9:58 am | Pisces | Water | Fruitful | 2nd |
| 18 Wed | Pisces | Water | Fruitful | 2nd |
| 19 Thu 12:58 pm | Aries | Fire | Barren | Full 7:13 am |
| 20 Fri | Aries | Fire | Barren | 3rd |
| 21 Sat 6:33 pm | Taurus | Earth | Semi-fruitful | 3rd |
| 22 Sun | Taurus | Earth | Semi-fruitful | 3rd |
| 23 Mon | Taurus | Earth | Semi-fruitful | 3rd |
| 24 Tue 3:34 am | Gemini | Air | Barren | 3rd |
| 25 Wed | Gemini | Air | Barren | 3rd |
| 26 Thu 3:24 pm | Cancer | Water | Fruitful | 4th 11:55 pm |
| 27 Fri | Cancer | Water | Fruitful | 4th |
| 28 Sat | Cancer | Water | Fruitful | 4th |
| 29 Sun 3:57 am | Leo | Fire | Barren | 4th |
| 30 Mon | Leo | Fire | Barren | 4th |

*Times are in Eastern Time.*

# October Moon Table

| Date | Sign | Element | Nature | Phase |
|------|------|---------|--------|-------|
| 1 Tue 2:52 pm | Virgo | Earth | Barren | 4th |
| 2 Wed | Virgo | Earth | Barren | 4th |
| 3 Thu 10:59 pm | Libra | Air | Semi-fruitful | 4th |
| 4 Fri | Libra | Air | Semi-fruitful | New 8:35 pm |
| 5 Sat | Libra | Air | Semi-fruitful | 1st |
| 6 Sun 4:33 am | Scorpio | Water | Fruitful | 1st |
| 7 Mon | Scorpio | Water | Fruitful | 1st |
| 8 Tue 8:21 am | Sagittarius | Fire | Barren | 1st |
| 9 Wed | Sagittarius | Fire | Barren | 1st |
| 10 Thu 11:17 am | Capricorn | Earth | Semi-fruitful | 1st |
| 11 Fri | Capricorn | Earth | Semi-fruitful | 2nd 7:02 pm |
| 12 Sat 2:00 pm | Aquarius | Air | Barren | 2nd |
| 13 Sun | Aquarius | Air | Barren | 2nd |
| 14 Mon 5:06 pm | Pisces | Water | Fruitful | 2nd |
| 15 Tue | Pisces | Water | Fruitful | 2nd |
| 16 Wed 9:18 pm | Aries | Fire | Barren | 2nd |
| 17 Thu | Aries | Fire | Barren | 2nd |
| 18 Fri | Aries | Fire | Barren | Full 7:38 pm |
| 19 Sat 3:27 am | Taurus | Earth | Semi-fruitful | 3rd |
| 20 Sun | Taurus | Earth | Semi-fruitful | 3rd |
| 21 Mon 12:14 pm | Gemini | Air | Barren | 3rd |
| 22 Tue | Gemini | Air | Barren | 3rd |
| 23 Wed 11:36 pm | Cancer | Water | Fruitful | 3rd |
| 24 Thu | Cancer | Water | Fruitful | 3rd |
| 25 Fri | Cancer | Water | Fruitful | 3rd |
| 26 Sat 12:12 pm | Leo | Fire | Barren | 4th 7:40 pm |
| 27 Sun | Leo | Fire | Barren | 4th |
| 28 Mon 11:45 pm | Virgo | Earth | Barren | 4th |
| 29 Tue | Virgo | Earth | Barren | 4th |
| 30 Wed | Virgo | Earth | Barren | 4th |
| 31 Thu 8:22 am | Libra | Air | Semi-fruitful | 4th |

*Times are in Eastern Time.*

# November Moon Table

| Date | Sign | Element | Nature | Phase |
|------|------|---------|--------|-------|
| 1 Fri | Libra | Air | Semi-fruitful | 4th |
| 2 Sat 1:35 pm | Scorpio | Water | Fruitful | 4th |
| 3 Sun | Scorpio | Water | Fruitful | New 7:50 am |
| 4 Mon 3:14 pm | Sagittarius | Fire | Barren | 1st |
| 5 Tue | Sagittarius | Fire | Barren | 1st |
| 6 Wed 4:44 pm | Capricorn | Earth | Semi-fruitful | 1st |
| 7 Thu | Capricorn | Earth | Semi-fruitful | 1st |
| 8 Fri 6:30 pm | Aquarius | Air | Barren | 1st |
| 9 Sat | Aquarius | Air | Barren | 1st |
| 10 Sun 9:36 pm | Pisces | Water | Fruitful | 2nd 12:57 am |
| 11 Mon | Pisces | Water | Fruitful | 2nd |
| 12 Tue | Pisces | Water | Fruitful | 2nd |
| 13 Wed 2:39 am | Aries | Fire | Barren | 2nd |
| 14 Thu | Aries | Fire | Barren | 2nd |
| 15 Fri 9:49 am | Taurus | Earth | Semi-fruitful | 2nd |
| 16 Sat | Taurus | Earth | Semi-fruitful | 2nd |
| 17 Sun 7:07 pm | Gemini | Air | Barren | Full 10:16 am |
| 18 Mon | Gemini | Air | Barren | 3rd |
| 19 Tue | Gemini | Air | Barren | 3rd |
| 20 Wed 6:23 am | Cancer | Water | Fruitful | 3rd |
| 21 Thu | Cancer | Water | Fruitful | 3rd |
| 22 Fri 6:56 pm | Leo | Fire | Barren | 3rd |
| 23 Sat | Leo | Fire | Barren | 3rd |
| 24 Sun | Leo | Fire | Barren | 3rd |
| 25 Mon 7:11 am | Virgo | Earth | Barren | 4th 2:28 pm |
| 26 Tue | Virgo | Earth | Barren | 4th |
| 27 Wed 5:00 pm | Libra | Air | Semi-fruitful | 4th |
| 28 Thu | Libra | Air | Semi-fruitful | 4th |
| 29 Fri 11:03 pm | Scorpio | Water | Fruitful | 4th |
| 30 Sat | Scorpio | Water | Fruitful | 4th |

*Times are in Eastern Time.*

# December Moon Table

| Date | Sign | Element | Nature | Phase |
|------|------|---------|--------|-------|
| 1 Sun | Scorpio | Water | Fruitful | 4th |
| 2 Mon 1:31 am | Sagittarius | Fire | Barren | New 7:22 pm |
| 3 Tue | Sagittarius | Fire | Barren | 1st |
| 4 Wed 1:49 am | Capricorn | Earth | Semi-fruitful | 1st |
| 5 Thu | Capricorn | Earth | Semi-fruitful | 1st |
| 6 Fri 1:53 am | Aquarius | Air | Barren | 1st |
| 7 Sat | Aquarius | Air | Barren | 1st |
| 8 Sun 3:34 am | Pisces | Water | Fruitful | 1st |
| 9 Mon | Pisces | Water | Fruitful | 2nd 10:12 am |
| 10 Tue 8:06 am | Aries | Fire | Barren | 2nd |
| 11 Wed | Aries | Fire | Barren | 2nd |
| 12 Thu 3:40 pm | Taurus | Earth | Semi-fruitful | 2nd |
| 13 Fri | Taurus | Earth | Semi-fruitful | 2nd |
| 14 Sat | Taurus | Earth | Semi-fruitful | 2nd |
| 15 Sun 1:40 am | Gemini | Air | Barren | 2nd |
| 16 Mon | Gemini | Air | Barren | 2nd |
| 17 Tue 1:17 pm | Cancer | Water | Fruitful | Full 4:28 am |
| 18 Wed | Cancer | Water | Fruitful | 3rd |
| 19 Thu | Cancer | Water | Fruitful | 3rd |
| 20 Fri 1:48 am | Leo | Fire | Barren | 3rd |
| 21 Sat | Leo | Fire | Barren | 3rd |
| 22 Sun 2:19 pm | Virgo | Earth | Barren | 3rd |
| 23 Mon | Virgo | Earth | Barren | 3rd |
| 24 Tue | Virgo | Earth | Barren | 3rd |
| 25 Wed 1:17 am | Libra | Air | Semi-fruitful | 4th 8:48 am |
| 26 Thu | Libra | Air | Semi-fruitful | 4th |
| 27 Fri 8:58 am | Scorpio | Water | Fruitful | 4th |
| 28 Sat | Scorpio | Water | Fruitful | 4th |
| 29 Sun 12:37 pm | Sagittarius | Fire | Barren | 4th |
| 30 Mon | Sagittarius | Fire | Barren | 4th |
| 31 Tue 1:01 pm | Capricorn | Earth | Semi-fruitful | 4th |

*Times are in Eastern Time.*

# Dates to Destroy Weeds and Pests

| From | | To | | Sign | Quarter |
|------|------|------|------|------|---------|
| Jan 8 | 3:28 am | Jan 10 | 3:54 am | Sagittarius | 4th |
| Jan 26 | 11:38 pm | Jan 28 | 6:27 pm | Leo | 3rd |
| Jan 28 | 6:27 pm | Jan 31 | 1:36 am | Virgo | 3rd |
| Feb 4 | 10:45 am | Feb 6 | 12:55 pm | Sagittarius | 4th |
| Feb 8 | 2:16 pm | Feb 10 | 2:20 am | Aquarius | 4th |
| Feb 25 | 3:26 pm | Feb 27 | 8:02 am | Virgo | 3rd |
| Mar 3 | 4:11 pm | Mar 4 | 4:53 pm | Sagittarius | 3rd |
| Mar 4 | 4:53 pm | Mar 5 | 7:14 pm | Sagittarius | 4th |
| Mar 7 | 10:01 pm | Mar 10 | 1:19 am | Aquarius | 4th |
| Mar 30 | 11:13 pm | Apr 2 | 1:35 am | Sagittarius | 3rd |
| Apr 4 | 4:41 am | Apr 6 | 9:00 am | Aquarius | 4th |
| Apr 8 | 3:02 pm | Apr 10 | 5:35 am | Aries | 4th |
| Apr 27 | 7:32 am | Apr 29 | 8:21 am | Sagittarius | 3rd |
| May 1 | 10:20 am | May 2 | 7:14 am | Aquarius | 3rd |
| May 2 | 7:14 am | May 3 | 2:25 pm | Aquarius | 4th |
| May 5 | 9:03 pm | May 8 | 6:09 am | Aries | 4th |
| May 25 | 12:25 am | May 26 | 5:28 pm | Sagittarius | 3rd |
| May 28 | 5:48 pm | May 30 | 8:30 pm | Aquarius | 3rd |
| Jun 2 | 2:33 am | Jun 4 | 11:53 am | Aries | 4th |
| Jun 6 | 11:32 pm | Jun 8 | 11:56 am | Gemini | 4th |
| Jun 25 | 3:27 am | Jun 27 | 4:32 am | Aquarius | 3rd |
| Jun 29 | 9:07 am | Jun 30 | 12:54 am | Aries | 3rd |
| Jun 30 | 12:54 am | Jul 1 | 5:43 pm | Aries | 4th |
| Jul 4 | 5:21 am | Jul 6 | 6:14 pm | Gemini | 4th |
| Jul 22 | 2:16 pm | Jul 24 | 2:22 pm | Aquarius | 3rd |
| Jul 26 | 5:29 pm | Jul 29 | 12:43 am | Aries | 3rd |

*Times are in Eastern Time.*

# Dates to Destroy Weeds and Pests

| From | | To | | Sign | Quarter |
|------|------|------|------|------|---------|
| Jul 31 | 11:42 am | Aug 3 | 12:29 am | Gemini | 4th |
| Aug 5 | 12:58 pm | Aug 6 | 5:51 pm | Leo | 4th |
| Aug 20 | 9:45 pm | Aug 21 | 12:43 am | Aquarius | 3rd |
| Aug 23 | 3:13 am | Aug 25 | 9:13 am | Aries | 3rd |
| Aug 27 | 7:08 pm | Aug 28 | 5:35 am | Gemini | 3rd |
| Aug 28 | 5:35 am | Aug 30 | 7:33 am | Gemini | 4th |
| Sep 1 | 8:01 pm | Sep 4 | 6:43 am | Leo | 4th |
| Sep 4 | 6:43 am | Sep 5 | 7:36 am | Virgo | 4th |
| Sep 19 | 12:58 pm | Sep 21 | 6:33 pm | Aries | 3rd |
| Sep 24 | 3:34 am | Sep 26 | 3:24 pm | Gemini | 3rd |
| Sep 29 | 3:57 am | Oct 1 | 2:52 pm | Leo | 4th |
| Oct 1 | 2:52 pm | Oct 3 | 10:59 pm | Virgo | 4th |
| Oct 18 | 7:38 pm | Oct 19 | 3:27 am | Aries | 3rd |
| Oct 21 | 12:14 pm | Oct 23 | 11:36 pm | Gemini | 3rd |
| Oct 26 | 12:12 pm | Oct 26 | 7:40 pm | Leo | 3rd |
| Oct 26 | 7:40 pm | Oct 28 | 11:45 pm | Leo | 4th |
| Oct 28 | 11:45 pm | Oct 31 | 8:22 am | Virgo | 4th |
| Nov 17 | 7:07 pm | Nov 20 | 6:23 am | Gemini | 3rd |
| Nov 22 | 6:56 pm | Nov 25 | 7:11 am | Leo | 3rd |
| Nov 25 | 7:11 am | Nov 25 | 2:28 pm | Virgo | 3rd |
| Nov 25 | 2:28 pm | Nov 27 | 5:00 pm | Virgo | 4th |
| Dec 2 | 1:31 am | Dec 2 | 7:22 pm | Sagittarius | 4th |
| Dec 17 | 4:28 am | Dec 17 | 1:17 pm | Gemini | 3rd |
| Dec 20 | 1:48 am | Dec 22 | 2:19 pm | Leo | 3rd |
| Dec 22 | 2:19 pm | Dec 25 | 1:17 am | Virgo | 3rd |
| Dec 29 | 12:37 pm | Dec 31 | 1:01 pm | Sagittarius | 4th |

*Times are in Eastern Time.*

# About the Authors

**Elizabeth Barrette** has been involved with the Pagan community for more than twenty-three years. She served as Managing Editor of *PanGaia* for eight years and Dean of Studies at the Grey School of Wizardry for four years. Her book *Composing Magic: How to Create Magical Spells, Rituals, Blessings, Chants, and Prayers* explains how to combine writing and spirituality. She enjoys magical crafts, historic religions, and gardening for wildlife. Visit her blog, *The Wordsmith's Forge* (http://ysabetwordsmith .livejournal.com), or her website, *PenUltimate Productions* (http:// penultimateproductions.weebly.com).

**Calantirniel** has practiced many forms of natural spirituality since the early 1990s. She is a professional astrologer, tarot card reader, dowser, flower essence creator and practitioner, and Usui Reiki Master and became a ULC Reverend and a Master Herbalist in 2007. She has an organic garden, crochets professionally, and is co-creating the spiritual path Tië eldaliéva, meaning "the Elven Path." Please visit http://astroherbalist.com for more information.

**Dallas Jennifer Cobb** lives a magical life, manifesting meaningful and flexible work, satisfying relationships, and abundant gardens. She enjoys a balance of time and money, which support her deepest desires: a loving family, time in nature, self-expression, and a healthy home. She lives in paradise, in a waterfront village in rural Ontario. Contact her at jennifer.cobb @live.com.

**Sally Cragin** is the author of *Born on the Cusp: Birthdays Between the Signs* and *The Astrological Elements*, both published by Llewellyn. She writes the "Moon Signs" forecasts for the *Boston Phoenix* and also sees clients in her astrology and tarot work. She teaches history and writing at Fitchburg (MA) State University, and serves on the Fitchburg School Committee.

**Alice DeVille** is an internationally known astrologer, writer, and metaphysical consultant. An accomplished cook, Alice enjoys preparing American, Italian, French, Tex-Mex, and Southern cuisine and enjoys creating new recipes. Well-known in the community for hosting buffet dinners for up to 200 guests during the holiday season, Alice would prepare 40 to 50 appetizers, side, main dishes, and desserts for a single five-hour affair. She is available for writing books and articles. Contact Alice at DeVilleAA@aol.com.

**Emyme** returned to earth-based beliefs several years ago, having dabbled as a teen. A solitary eclectic, she creates magick through writing, gardening, crafts, and the domestic arts of cooking and baking. Her home, Das Haus von schönen Frauen ("the house of beautiful women"), is multigenerational and multi-cat; and embodies Maiden/Mother/Crone. She is the author of *The Splendid, Blended Family*, a children's picture book about step-families and holidays. Contact catsmeow24 @verizon.net for news of her website and blog.

**Darcey Blue French** trained as a clinical herbalist and nutritionist at the North American Institute of Medical Herbalism under Paul Bergner. It is her deep love of the wild earth and its creatures that fuels her passion for healing and teaching about plants, wilderness, spirit, nourishment, and healing. Learn more about her at www.blueturtlebotanicals.blogspot.com.

**Jill Henderson** is an artist, author, and world traveler with a penchant for wild edible and medicinal plants and nature ecology. She writes and edits the weekly blog *Show Me Oz* (http://showmeoz.wordpress.com) and is the author of three books: *The Healing Power of Kitchen Herbs*, *A Journey of Seasons*, and *The Garden Seed Saving Guide*. In her spare time, Jill presents seed saving workshops and creates professional pet portraits and wildlife art (http://foreverpetportraits.word press.com). She and her husband, Dean, live in the heart of the rugged Ozark Mountains.

**JD Hortwort** resides in North Carolina. She is an avid student of herbology and gardening, a professional writer, and an award-winning journalist.

**Cindy Jones, Ph.D.**, is a biochemist, herbalist, and farmer who works as a cosmetic formulator of natural skin care products. She owns Sagescript Institute, LLC, a company that provides botanical/herbal ingredients, consults on product development, and provides education in the area of cosmetics and herbs. She also produces the Colorado Aromatics brand of skin care products. She lives with her family and animals on their farm in Colorado. Visit her website at http://www.sagescript.com and her blog at http://sagescript.blogspot.com.

**James Kambos** is an herbalist, writer, and artist from Ohio. He raises a wide variety of herbs and perennials in his small garden. His interest in herbs began as a child when he became captivated by the scent and beauty of the herbs his grandmother raised in her kitchen garden. He enjoys preserving and cooking with herbs. A regular contributor to Llewellyn's annuals, he also enjoys incorporating the magical energy of herbs into spellcrafting.

**Lisa Mc Sherry** lives outside of Seattle with her husband, dog, and two cats. Cancer-free since late 2009, she runs a review site, FacingNorth.net, and more of her writing is on her website, cybercoven.org.

**Lexa Olick** is the author of *Witchy Crafts: 60 Enchanted Projects for the Creative Witch*, forthcoming from Llewellyn in winter 2013. She is also an artist, writer, silversmith, and teacher and holds degrees in both art and art history. She participates in art shows around New York and is always happy to share her passion for art and writing with others.

**Susan Pesznecker, M.S.**, is a child of the natural world and a student of astronomy, herbology, healing, stonework, green magicks, and folklore. A degreed writer, Sue teaches writing and literature at two local universities and teaches magick in the online Grey School (www.greyschool.com). She is the author of *Gargoyles* (New Page), *Crafting Magick with Pen and Ink* (Llewellyn), and the forthcoming *The Magickal Retreat: Making Time for Solitude, Intention, and Rejuvenation* (Llewellyn). You can contact Sue through her Facebook page or her website, www.susanpesznecker.com.

**Kelly Proudfoot,** originally from Australia, now lives in Nashville, Tennessee, and is interested in magical herbalism, mythology, dream therapy, and quantum mechanics. She's been a practicing numerologist and tarot reader for twenty years. She is in the process of setting up her herb farm and Wiccan supply business.

**Linda Raedisch** is the author of *Night of the Witches: Folklore, Traditions and Recipes for Celebrating Walpurgis Night* and a frequent contributor to Llewellyn's annuals. She lives in northern

New Jersey where Spitzenbergs and Sheep's Nose apples have historically been grown, and where a particularly thorny variety of *Malus coronaria* continues to flourish.

**Charlie Rainbow Wolf** is of Cherokee and English heritage and has studied the mysteries of both cultures. She is a practitioner of shamanic healing, crystal therapy, and meditation as medicine. She is a member of the ATA, is certified as a professional reader by the TCBA, works as an intuitive adviser for a prestigious international company, and is the Dean of Faculty and a teacher at the Grey School of Wizardry. She is keenly interested in pottery, soapmaking, and organic gardening.

**Suzanne Ress** has been writing fiction and nonfiction for over twenty-five years. She is an accomplished, self-taught herb gardener, beekeeper, silversmith, and mosaicist. She lives at the foot of the Alps in northern Italy with her husband, daughter, three dogs, three horses, and many wild animals.

**Laurel Reufner's** mother can verify that she grew up a "wild child" in farming country. Laurel has been earth-centered for over twenty years now and really enjoys writing about topics that grab her attention. Laurel has always lived in Southeastern Ohio and currently calls Athens County home, where she lives with her wonderful husband and two wild children of her own. Visit her website at http://laurelreufner.blogspot.com.

**Anne Sala** is a freelance journalist and mother. She currently resides in Minnesota, where she tends a finicky potted bay tree that really dislikes the cold.

**Carole Schwalm** lives in Sante Fe, New Mexico. She has contributed to self-help articles and writes for America Online and other websites.